This book is dedicated to:

Everyone one of you that has ever felt lost in their skin,
felt like the right mind in the wrong body,

and everyone that is in need of a helping hand.

The only thing left to lose now is your doubt.

- Carrie -

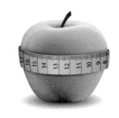

CR NUTRITION

FRESH START RESET

The 14-day Bariatric Body and Mind Reset

For your Pouch or Sleeve

Author

Holistic Nutritionist and Bariatric Health Coach

Carrie-Anne Ross

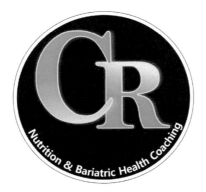

http://www.crnutrition.net

Third Ed. Fresh Start Reset ©2018 CR Nutrition and Bariatric Health Coaching

Second Ed. The Fresh Start Pouch Reset©2017 CR Nutrition and Bariatric Health Coaching

First Ed. Bariatric Keto Reset©2017 CR Nutrition and Bariatric Health Coaching

Content provided in this book is of a general supplemental nature and does not replace the information and advice provided by your own health care professionals but may be used in addition to your current health care plan. CR Nutrition does not endorse the cessation of any prescribed medications. Always consult **YOUR** own health providers for specific personal health and medical advice or to see if a program is right for you.

FRESH START RESET

Introduction

Making the connection between your brain and your body can be one of the most difficult things to do, second to admitting that you need help and asking for it.

You took the plunge and had weight loss surgery. You are a 'sleever', or a 'bypasser'. You have had a band, or the Duodenal switch. What ever your surgery type, you took a chance and put your faith in the surgeon and their plan for you.

Your doctors and surgeons all tell you that the surgery is going to be your tool for weight loss and give you expectations of an amount that you need to lose per visit. You follow your plan, and the weight comes of a little at first and a little more, but it isn't the same as other people, it is actually a lot harder than you anticipated. Part of your stomach is removed but all of the challenges and negative thoughts remain.

Now you have a different set of mental struggles, why aren't you losing weight? Why is it falling off the last person, the next person and the one after, but not you?

Did they even do this surgery at all? Why did I bother?

Does it seem like your thoughts are the things that should have been operated on instead of your stomach?

You never lost the amount of weight you wanted to, or you reached your goal only to hover there for the briefest of time just to start gaining again. It's a few years down the track and you have regained half of what you lost. It's your second surgical anniversary and you realise that you can now eat double the portions that you could a year ago. What is going on?

There are so many things that need to be addressed in weight loss and weight loss surgery in order to give us the best possible outcomes in recovery. This is something that we don't all receive in the 10 minute post-surgical follow ups. So it is up to us to make the connections between our mind, our bodies and our health.

The Art Of Mindfulness

Why do we need to be mindful?

Sometimes we feel that our journey and our progress should be further along than it is, leading us to feelings of low self worth, self depreciation, anger, resentful of the successes of others and frustration. It is so difficult to be patient when you have wanted something so desperately your whole life, but success takes time.

Quick found results are undone just as quickly, as you have not allowed yourself to truly adopt and adapt to change. You add stress and pressure to yourself to achieve 'something', not recognising or giving credit to the steps you have taken thus far. You get down on yourself and place negative impact on your mental health, which holds more pieces to the puzzle than you realise. You stop yourself succeeding by focussing on why you haven't yet reached your ultimate goal.

Unfortunately, your surgery is not the issue here, it is you.

Now this isn't permission to 'blame' yourself for anything, it is simply a prompt for you to recognise the impact you have on your own success and change your behaviour.

This is where mindfulness plays a huge part, and we are going to explore why.

Being Mindful

Reconnecting with Self

When you look at other people, you see qualities that you may judge or overvalue. This is human nature. We have a natural affinity for people who possess values we admire and wish to have for ourselves, and conversely , tend to avoid those whose traits contradict our own values.

What we are failing to recognise in this process is that those traits that we value and admire, are traits that our true selves possess. This is why you need to reconnect with these values so that you can truly focus on becoming the 'you' that you value. You will learn to value yourself.

So, think about yourself in terms of traits. You have been floating in a certain mindset for so long that you have allowed certain parts of your psyche to become the dominant traits. What are they?

Are you the carer? The one who is always taking care of others to the point that they neglect themselves.

Are you the negative friend? The 'Debbie Downer'? The one who just cannot seem to find joy in any situation and always has a bad thought or feeling about it?

Are you the Avoider? Do you decline social engagements more often than not?

Are you the stressor? Withdrawn Partner? Depressed Mother? Jealous Girlfriend? Resentful weight loser?

Which part of you have you allowed to become dominant through the years of being overweight and unhealthy. Is this dominant personality trait something that you value or admire?

What about the traits that you don't value? What do you do about them ?

These can be a useful tool in rediscovering who YOU are. For example, you dislike or are intolerant of loud noises, this indicates that your core self is predominantly of a quiet or subdued nature and that you value being calm. Do you have a distaste for selfishness? Well then your core personality trait is that you are of a generous nature. You need to identify what traits you dislike, and use them to identify your positive characteristics.

Make a list and use it to reconnect with YOU.

The traits or actions I dislike are...	This means I am a person who is ...
Example: Cheating partner	Loyal and value my relationships

Now look over your list… Who are YOU?

Mindful Eating

Reframing your food thinking

Mindfulness is an effective cognitive behavioural therapy approach to changing an individuals negative or damaging behaviours. It encourages awareness, not only of environment but also of self. Mindfulness helps to put you in touch with the thoughts and feelings that have a tendency to dictate actions.

To be mindful, you have to make yourself 'present'. What does that mean?

It means showing up to your own emotion party. It means being there in the moment and recognising it for what it is. JUST A FEELING. It means not running to the fridge or pantry to hide from negative situations.

Being mindful, or being present in the feeling allows you to recognise the feeling for what it is, and that is, "just a feeling". Identifying these feelings can be the answer to why you have a tendency to overeat, or why you find it difficult to lose weight.

You'll be able to figure out the reasons behind your actions.

Is your eating simply a responsive action due to:

- The negative feelings associated with confrontation?

- Anxiety caused by stress in the workplace?

- Feelings of low self worth?

- Wanting to celebrate a good feeling?

The majority of the time, the answer will be yes. But, the question should really be, 'How can you overcome or enjoy these feelings **without** food'?

The answer is mindfulness. Mindfulness puts you ahead of the situation to act as gatekeeper to actions. Mindfulness allows you to ask the questions that will either allow or deny any action from being derived from a feeling.

Mindfulness is stopping the feeling in its tracks and questioning its intention.

You are *'craving'* chocolate, of course you can have a piece of chocolate, you are after all an adult. But before you do, ask yourself,

- Do you REALLY want it?

- Do you REALLY NEED it?

- Do you really FEEL like it right now?

- Can it wait?

- Will chocolate etc., really resolve the issue I am faced with?"

Mindfulness helps us pause in the moment to question our own intention with aim to diffuse actions that have a negative impact on ourselves. It helps you to develop and put into place, mechanisms that help you cope with emotion and to reframe potentially damaging patterns of thinking.

Mindfulness helps you pull the plug on negative self talk as you diffuse the thoughts before they have time to charge your actions. You will learn to stop comparing yourself to others and their journeys, that their experience is exactly that, **THEIRS**

Mindful eating helps you take notice of your habits and prevents you from:

- Eating too quickly to recognize when you are satisfied.

- Not eating balanced meals.

- Drinking too soon before, during or after eating.

- Not eating your proteins first.

- Skipping meals, and allowing hunger to dictate poor choices.

- Having 'one more bite' or 'just a little bit more'

MINDFUL EATING TIPS

Eat dense protein as it will make you feel fuller and keep you satiated for longer. For example; beef, chicken or shrimp instead of cheese and eggs. Also, it would be more beneficial to ditch the protein shakes and have dense wholefood protein sources instead.

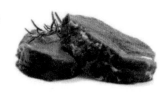

Grass-fed Organic is always best, but buy what you can afford as Meat based protein is an excellent source of Haem-Iron. A vital micronutrient for all our vital functions. Bariatric patients have an increased need for both protein and Iron.

Be prepared for situations that will challenge you. You can do this by taking a snack bag of parmesan crisps, cheese, meat or nuts in your purse when you go to a gathering where you'll know you will be faced with temptation.

Eat 'time consuming foods'. For instance; 10 unshelled pistachios have an average of 30 calories, 2g carbohydrate and 1g protein. This would be a great snack for those of you who

'aren't sure whether or not they are hungry'.

By the time it takes to shell and eat each nut, you'll soon have conquered your cravings for less healthy options. Plus, you get a tasty little savoury snack.

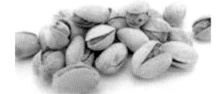

Pistachios contain fewer calories and more potassium and vitamin K per serving than other nuts. There is also research to suggest that that are have the ability to lower cholesterol and help in blood sugar regulation.

Have a schedule and stick to it. Know that at 11am you are going to have protein and salad. Know that at 1pm you have a snack. Know at 1:30pm you have a glass of water. Know your direction.

- Use the tools you have to your best benefit. This means using your tracker app (such as My Fitness Pal), to LOG EVERYTHING. Feel free to use any tracker that you like, it is always about what works for you.

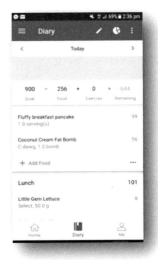

- Get to know your quantities so you know them from sight alone, know what a portion is. You can take pictures of your portions on your phone and refer back to them when needed, or print them and stick them to your fridge.

- Plan your day of eating ahead of time. By doing this, you'll know where you are headed, and know how to rearrange your day to fit in that low-carb pudding at the end of the day (if you want to have one and it fits into your plan *Balanced Macros©). .

- Remember your limitations and act accordingly. You KNOW you can't have that one more bite, you KNOW you can't sit in front of the TV and gorge on crisps.

- Remembering how far you've come and what got you here in the first place should be in the forefront of every food choice you make. This is not to make you fear food, or to make you feel guilty, but rather to keep you mindful of your level of control over ALL of your choices.

- If you are lucky enough to engage is a social group , whether this be on the internet or in person, draw on the strength of its members for   guidance and support.

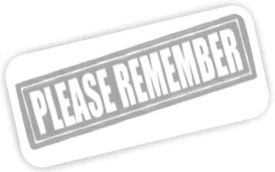

Committing yourself to change

When you begin any program, you initially need to commit your mind to change. You need to ensure that your mental toolkit is full of all the tools you will need to achieve your success.

One of the main tools for success that you need to make accessible to yourself is support. It is of the utmost importance that you are aware of who your supports are and how to access them.

Support networks are the people that you have on hand to help you through your struggles. They may be friends, family or even a social media group like the CR Nutrition and Bariatric Heath Coaching Group page. They can be internet based forums of likeminded and like-goaled individuals, all eager to help you reach your highest potentials. These are the people that are going to fill you with confidence when you are feeling doubtful. They are the ones that will remind you of your strength to overcome challenges of willpower. These are the people to whom you will express your fears of failure, and they very same people that will get you through to the next day. So you need to access and utilise this most valuable resource and also give it back when you can.

Never be afraid to ask for help. Someone else may just have enough strength to give you the boost you need to get you through to the next day. You can then reciprocate and help them when they need it. That is how support works.

So join the likeminded people in your group forums and do not be afraid to say

"I am human and I feel like my willpower is being challenged, who else feels like this is a tough goal to achieve?"

You will soon realise that you are not alone and there is immense strength and support in numbers. SO, REMEMBER… Reach out for help and to help others. Sometimes giving others strength has a trickle back effect and will help you cement your own resolve.

Planning and Preparation

You have to be prepared for success to make it stick. Being prepared is one of the most important aspects and a vital 'key' to success. But what does that entail? It means knowing where you are going and exactly how you are going to get there. So,

Plan your meals: Know what you are going to eat and when you are going to eat it. This is going to help you avoid and manage any tendency to overeat. Scheduling your meals also helps to ensure that you do not go hungry and that your energy stores are sustained throughout the day. This also includes logging your meals in your preferred meal tracking app (i.e. My Fitness Pal). Having a plan is going to help you avoid any hunger driven bad food choices.

Research your recipes and know your portions sizes: You know what your intake capacity should be, so only serve yourself that much and log that much in your app, and incorporate your mindfulness practices to stay true to that knowledge. Keep your path to success clear and straight by making your plan fool proof.

Ask, ask and ask again: Draw on the expertise and experience of your fellow 'sleevers'etc; successful losers and your peers. Ask questions until you know all the answers. Don't fly blind, you need to have all your bases covered, and arm yourself against excuses of ignorance to the facts.

Use your support networks: Don't be afraid to ask for help, that is why they are there .

Always be mindful: Always stay truthful to yourself. Don't play the old tune of " I always eat the right things, and I follow my plan 100% but still cannot lose, if you know full well that there are things that you don't do correctly.

You have to make yourself present in your process and be truthful to yourself. No one is going to hold you accountable for your actions (or lack of action), but you. Healing and relearning are a constant process that require and deserve your full attention.

Focus on one goal at a time: multitasking isn't the answer. A divided and exhausted brain is going to lead you down the wrong path where old habits hide. You need to stay mindful and resist distractions. Set boundaries for yourself and others. This is how you are going to achieve your goals.

Aim to achieve realistic goals. When you gain this focus you gain control.

What are your realistic goals?

Reasonable Goal	How will I achieve it?	By When?
i.e. Reset my satiety point	By doing the pouch reset	14 days and ongoing

Understanding the Physical

Is it possible to have a Fresh Start and Reset my Pouch?

There are literally handfuls of 'pouch reset' plans floating around on the internet. They promote themselves as being able to physically shrink the size of your stomach pouch (the small pouch like stomach that was created for you during your surgery). They claim to be able to give you back your restrictions and shrink your pouch to post-surgical size. Ironically, the term 'shrink' is used a little too loosely. The truth of the matter is, you cannot 'shrink' your stomach in physical size.

Your stomach is made up of a multi-folded muscular membrane that expands and contracts as part of digestion. These folds are called rugae.

The folds, or rugae, are there to allow expansion and contraction to happen, and it is thought that this was how the human body adapted through times of famine and feasting. During famine the stomach rugae would contract tightly in the absence of food, giving the stomach a smaller volume and therefore inducing the feeling of fullness or satiety from less food. Then in times of abundance, would allow larger more frequent amounts of food to be consumed, stretching the stomach to full capacity. In todays world, we seem to be living in times of constant excess, which has seemingly resulted in the obesity crisis that we face. The stomachs of so many have become accustomed to a lifetime of abundance , and their rugae never have a chance to contract back, instead learn to stretch and accommodate more.

An analogy for this process is, the weight lifter.

A weight lifter trains regularly to get his muscles used to lifting a certain level of weights. The more he lifts, and the more often he lifts it, the more used to it he becomes until he decides to add more weight.

Well the same is true for the stomach. The more food you eat, and the more often you eat it, the more used to this quantity your stomach will become.

The unfortunate side of this analogy is that whilst the weightlifter increases his strength, the eater increases their waistline.

However, if that same weight lifter decided to only lift half of his average for a set period of time, he would soon find himself accustomed to the lower weight. His overall capacity for lifting will not have changed, but his ability to lift his maximum will have been decreased. His muscles will have become used to doing less work.

So if the weight lifter decides to only lift half of his average for a time, what do you think will happen if one day he decided to try and lift the total again? That's right, he will struggle, and this is because his muscles have 'learned' to do less work.

The same can be said for our stomachs, and this ability remains, even after surgery. So while you cannot physically "shrink your stomach', what you can do is **reset your satiety point**. What that means is that you can reconfigure the point at which fullness is signalled without overdoing it and without overeating. You can retrain your stomach to want less.

This plan is going to help you reset your 'maximum lifting capacity' and you are going to retrain your mind and body to eat less.

There are so many plans, so what makes this one successful?

Well, quite simply, it addresses the important factors that contribute to your current health states. As mentioned, there are hundreds of pouch reset plans that claim to shrink your pouch in as little as 3-5 days. One might have to wonder, is 3-5 days adequate to address the long standing and deeply rooted associations and poor decisions about food? I don't think that's possible. This plan does not try to convince you that such important preparation and change can be completed in such a trivial time frame. Lets be honest with ourselves, we wouldn't be looking at a Fresh Start Pouch Reset if we didn't need additional time and support.

In honesty, if we were able to fix these issues in a few days, we probably wouldn't have ended up on the operating table to begin with. Am I right?

This Fresh Start Pouch Reset program is a methodical and structured transitional program that gives you a new start and the building blocks to take you further into ongoing weight loss and goal weight maintenance.

What makes this different again is that you will not be required to succumb to a post surgical diet plan of baby food like mush. These foods are recommended to promote gentle digestive processes while your post-operative stomach is healing. There are no products or shakes being peddled. Replacing all your meals with protein shakes is not helping you address your issues with food. This practice is simply exchanging one set of disordered eating practices with another extreme way of eating, and nothing more than clever marketing by companies who make money off your vulnerability.

Honestly it seems strange to try and combat issues with food by restricting yourself to puree or protein shakes. Wouldn't you agree?

The Fresh Start Program asks you to be honest and realistic. To set clear and achievable goals. To be mindful of, and accountable for your choices, and it offers real food choices in a proper manageable structure.

It asks you to approach food in a new , honest and open way without having to restrict everything you eat and do. The Fresh Start Pouch Reset gives you mental and nutritional guidance through the tough processes and offers online forum support by the very same nutritionist that developed it. You are given a hand to get to your feet, then it is up to you to take the leap.

This is your chance to Eat to Succeed!!

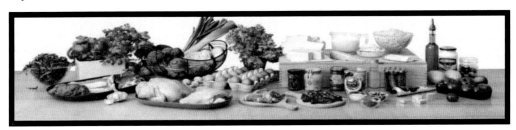

Metabolic Syndrome and Metabolic Resistance
Common Metabolic Syndrome and Metabolic Resistance questions

What is metabolic syndrome and how do I know if I have it?
How can I eat so little and NOT lose weight, sometimes I even GAIN?!!

Losing weight is a phenomenal feeling, it boosts self esteem, confidence and can change our whole lives for the better. However, we become comfortable with our eating practices and slowly but surely excess and over consumption begin to creep in again. When we are confident, we go out more, socialize more and do more. But we also find ourselves, eating more, drinking more and sleeping less. Before long we experience regain.

When we reduce our caloric intake our bodies adapt. This 'adaptation' changes our Basal Metabolic Rate (BMR — the caloric need at minimum to perform our vital functions at rest). When BMR lowers, the body adapts to run on less, which is why we stall. You may think that by lowering your intake and by eating so little that you will inevitably lose weight, but just like the weight lifter analogy, your body has learned to run on less. The problem is, we can not keep lowering intake to keep the losses going, what we must do is kick start the metabolisms to need more.

When stalls occur, this is signal to us that something needs changing, and the most important thing to remember is, it is about what we CAN (but aren't currently eating and doing) not what we can further cut out. Change usually requires the addition of something rather than the subtraction of something. So 'diets' are definitely NOT the answer. Diets restrict you, restrict your life, restrict your experiences and restrict you from being human. Diets lead to feelings of deprivation and resentment and ultimately "binge eating blow outs". When there is a fixation on what you CAN NOT have, you will be setting yourself up for failure. As humans, we ALL want what we cannot have.

You need to be focussing on getting your metabolism firing again. There are some things we can do after your reset, that can help that.

Metabolism Boosting, how to?

Don't skip meals

We want that metabolism burning bright and at its peak, so your body needs to know that it will be getting a constant supply of fuel. Skipping meals can slow your metabolism (this is the same for intermittent fasting which is not recommended for metabolic resistant people).

Eat at regular intervals

Again, metabolism boosting! Regular energy supply means your body wont hold onto what you are putting in. Aim to have your meal or snacks every 2-3 hours to keep blood sugar stable.

Don't Grab on the Go

Prepare proper nutritious foods and snacks. You don't want to put the wrong fuel in your gas tank, so try not to put the wrong fuel in you.

Get adequate sleep

Getting regular restorative sleep of approximately 7-8 hours a night is proven to keep your metabolic fires lit. Poor or irregular sleep will lead to disruption in hunger and satiety signalling (Ghrelin vs Leptin response) and lead you to snack!

Don't limit your calories drastically

As bariatric patients, your intake is substantially decreased, however the more you limit, the more your resistance will be ingrained. You need to aim for your 'sweet spot'. If you exercise, your intake will need to be increased also. In many cases your intake after surgery should be at around 1000-1200 calories a day by 12 months out of surgery, for continuous weight loss. With the aim being 1200 calories minimum from 12 months post op onwards.

Get some exercise

Regularly partaking in exercise, gentle or otherwise will help keep your metabolism chugging along. If you feel hungry after exercise, that's a good signal that your met-rate is being triggered.

Drink your Water

Ensure you get your minimum 64 oz. / 2 litres of water per day.

What about Ketosis?

Ketosis is a normal metabolic process that, in the absence of adequate glucose (sugar/ carbohydrate) in the diet, initiates fat utilisation instead. It does this by breaking down fats into fatty acids called ketones; which can be used in the absence of glucose to fuel its essential processes.

The body will begin to initiate the stages of ketosis when carbohydrate intake is limited, your glucose stores will be used until exhausted then the body will look to fat for fuel.

Ketosis can be achieved by regularly and consistently reducing your carbohydrate intake to under 50g per day, and is quite often maintained with intakes of under 75g a day consistently.

So there is NO NEED to drastically reduce your carbohydrate intake to levels as low as 20g per day. This level was designed and is prescribed for children with severe epilepsy. As adults, our needs are increased. Limiting your carbohydrate so low can have many negative effects, especially in those that have disorders relating to mental health, auto-immune, adrenal insufficiency or endocrine disruption. So be cautious of any plan that advocates 20g or less for all clients despite their individual health factors.

So, in short, by moderately (not drastically) reducing your carbohydrate intake, you can induce ketosis and start burning fat for fuel.

Why do we want to encourage Ketosis?

Metabolic Syndrome and Metabolic resistance usually go hand in hand with improper glucose vs insulin regulation. A large percentage of weight loss surgery participants have elevated and uncontrolled blood glucose levels and suffer for glycaemic events such as hypoglycaemia. The majority of obese or overweight individuals will have learned to act responsively to insulin production, and reach for the carbs when they are feeling low. This is how our 'sugar addicts' are created.

To enable us to re-regulate these mechanisms, we should first cover the basics.

- Carbohydrates cause a high-level insulin response, proteins cause a moderate level insulin response, and fats cause little to no insulin response.

- Insulin has a job. It is released in the presence of glucose and directs it where it needs to go. Removing it from the blood either to fuel bodily processes OR help store it away for later use. When glucose is in excess – it gets stored in the muscles and liver as 'glycogen' and can be released and converted back into glucose when needed via a process called Gluconeogenesis 'glu-co-neo-gen-esis'(which translates roughly to 'new sugar creation').

- The more carbohydrate we ingest, the more insulin we produce. But, eventually insulin release will STOP doing what it is supposed to, which is remove glucose from our blood. This means that blood glucose remains at elevated levels. This is called Type 2 Diabetes.

- When you are used to this level of carbohydrate vs insulin interaction, you WILL CRAVE carbohydrates when beginning a ketogenic style of eating. It's your bodies signalling process to tell you your glucose (main fuel supply) is running low. It will do this until you start utilizing fat. You need to retrain your insulin response and that can only do that by decreasing the carbohydrate level it is used to responding to.

- By lowering the insulin response, we can lower and control our blood sugar. This is because insulin isn't triggering stored glycogen to be released back into the system. This will diminish sugar cravings.

- Studies have shown ketogenic diets to be an excellent tool for managing, and in a lot of cases, reversing Type 2 Diabetes. Hypoglycaemic events are reduced if not eliminated when conforming to a low-carbohydrate dietary protocol. Further to this, studies are being conducted into its use in cancer treatment due to the nature of some 'sugar-feeding' cancers.

- Ketosis – Utilising fat as fuel. When we eat moderate amounts of fat, we breakdown our ingested fats into usable sources such as 'ketones'. If our dietary fat is insufficient and we need more to fuel the body, fat is released from its stores.

- This process happens very quickly and may seem at times that it isn't working. This is because the rapid emptying of cells results in them being filled with cellular fluid (water) as a 'space saver'. When your cells are called upon again to provide fat for fuel, the retained fluid is released. This is how many people can report periods of rapid weight loss. Many Keto sites call this the "whoosh".

- Fat is required for proper nervous system function, and is essential in the production of hormones.

- With the regulation of blood sugar, Ketosis helps to promote hormonal regulation resulting in better patterns of sleep, stabilisation of mood and has shown positive impact on menstrual symptom regulation.

- Fat is important for the absorption and utilisation of certain vitamins, to which deficiency has been linked to obesity and its comorbid states.

For instance, Vitamin D is a 'Fat-Soluble Vitamin'. This means that fat is used as a transport and carrier mechanism. Vitamin D is essential for immune function, for mental health, for bone growth and maintenance, as it aids in the absorption of calcium, and also essential in reproductive health. Fat ensures that we give certain vitamins the right vehicle for delivery.

WHY ENCOURAGE KETOSIS?

Not only to lose the weight, but also to gain better overall health by balancing blood sugar, hormonal regulation and boosting immune function. With a limited insulin response, you will have a lowered amount of free flowing insulin to demand sugar, and this also diminishes its capacity to store sugar.
Your sugar fuel light won't be flashing as it does in a hypoglycaemic episode, you'll be more balanced because you have adequate intake and adequate stores of fats.

HOW LONG DOES IT TAKE?

By reducing your carbohydrate intake to 50g or under in a consistent and stable manner, the glucose stores for the average person will be depleted in approximately 4-5 days. At this time you may experience what is referred to as Keto-flu.

During this 'keto flu' you might experience headaches, mild flu like symptoms, lethargy and general malaise. Best way to combat this is getting electrolytes which you can get by drinking bone broth, Propel or PowerAde zero, however try to avoid sweet tasting drinks on reset, artificially sweetened or otherwise. If you are suffering a headache, you can take pain relief. There is no need to suffer. You may also experience a change in body odour, breath and smelly urine/faeces. This is because of the change in diet, but signals that ketosis is actually happening. In time the breath and odour changes will lessen.

Several studies have been performed proving the efficacy of a ketogenic or con-trolled low carbohydrate diet, in the improvement of glycaemic control; and given the reduction of glycaemic fluctuation events such as hypo-glycaemia; even proven to aid in the reduction or cessation of taking glycaemia medications for Type 2 Diabetes. Providing evidence that lifestyle modification using low carbohydrate inter-ventions is effective for improving and reversing type 2 diabetes.

What about ketone strips? Should I get them?

Don't waste your time and money buying ketone testing strips, there is no such thing and no such levels of being in 'mild', 'moderate' or 'deep 'ketosis. Its more like a pregnancy test, you either are, or you aren't - the intensity of the pink line doesn't matter , if its there, its positive. Your reset is structured in such a way that you **will** achieve ketosis. After you complete the reset, you have the choice to move on and do the Balanced Macros Bariatric Ketogenic Plan ©, which will set you up with your own individually calculated macros to follow to help you maintain ketosis and continue your weight loss.

What about Exogenous Ketones? Am I upping my game and going to get into ketosis quicker?

No. *Exo-Ketones*, are another marketed idea in the weight loss and fitness in-dustry. What we must understand is that Ketones are the energy bi-product of the breakdown of dietary (or stored) fats. Ketones are the fuel that our cells need to run when in Ketosis, **they are NOT what breaks down the fat**.

Your body will utilise some for its energy needs and **you will expel the remaining**, and if your in the pee-stick crowd, you'll think that you are in keto-sis, when in fact you are literally pi**ing your money down the drain. Ketone supplements can however give you an energy boost, may curb hunger and have been anecdotally reported to enhance focus. But as for the proof on their efficacy in weight loss, the jury is still out. So if anyone is recommending them for weight loss, you might want to ask "**which ones are YOU SELLING**"?

What about Protein?

Be SMARTER not HARDER

There's lots of misinformation out there about what's the right amount of protein to be eating. Unfortunately the majority of this information comes from the fitness world and isn't regularly fact checked. If you want correct figures you need to look science.

Studies have calculated that the average human being (that's both men and women) require only 60g of protein per day to maintain lean muscle mass at goal weight. But you can get a little more specific, and calculate your own macros.

What's the calculation?

Our protein requirement is classified as the minimum daily protein intake to maintain lean body mass at your medically/ scientifically determined healthy body weight. Well lets start with YOUR minimum. Your medically ideal body weight as calculated by your height vs build is generally within a range.

Females																		
Height Ft	5'	5'1"	5'2"	5'3"	5'4"	5'5"	5'6"	5'7"	5'8"	5'9"	5'10"	5'11"	6'	6'1"	6'2"	6'3"	6'4"
Height cm	152	155	157	160	163	165	168	170	173	175	178	180	183	185	188	190	193
Ideal BW	45	48	50.	53	55	57	60	63	65	67	69	71	74	76	79	81	83
Max BW	58	60	62	64	66	68	71	75	78	79	82	85	88	90	94	97	99
Males																		
Height Ft	5'	5'1"	5'2"	5'3"	5'4"	5'5"	5'6"	5'7"	5'8"	5'9"	5'10"	5'11"	6'	6'1"	6'2"	6'3"	6'4"
Height cm	152	155	157	160	163	165	168	170	173	175	178	180	183	185	188	190	193
Ideal BW	53	55	57	59	61	63	65	67	69	71	73	75	78	80	83	85	87
Max BW	65	68	70	72	74	76	78	80	83	85	88	90	94	96	98	101	104

Table 1: Ideal Body weight range in **kilograms** – your weight can fall anywhere within the ideal to maximum body weight ranges
Please note that these tables are for a guide to calculate minimum protein ONLY and do not take muscle mass and build into account.

Females																	
Height Ft	5'	5'1"	5'2"	5'3"	5'4"	5'5"	5'6"	5'7"	5'8"	5'9"	5'10"	5'11"	6'	6'1"	6'2"	6'3"	6'4"
Height cm	152	155	157	160	163	165	168	170	173	175	178	180	183	185	188	190	193
Ideal BW	105	112	120	128	133	140	145	152	158	162	167	170	175	180	185	190	195
Max BW	125	135	140	145	150	155	160	165	170	175	180	185	190	195	200	205	210
Males																	
Height Ft	5'	5'1"	5'2"	5'3"	5'4"	5'5"	5'6"	5'7"	5'8"	5'9"	5'10"	5'11"	6'	6'1"	6'2"	6'3"	6'4"
Height cm	152	155	157	160	163	165	168	170	173	175	178	180	183	185	188	190	193
Ideal	115	120	125	133	140	147	152	160	168	175	181	188	195	200	205	210	215
Max BW	130	135	140	148	155	162	167	175	185	190	200	210	220	225	230	235	240

*Table 2: Ideal weight in **Pounds** – your weight can fall anywhere within the ideal to maximum body weight ranges . *Please note that these tables are for a guide to calculate minimum protein ONLY and do not take muscle mass and build into account.*

So, Lets say for example 70kg.

From that 70kg, we now have to subtract non lean mass. To do this we have to look at fat mass, if they are within their healthy range of 20- 25% Body fat for women, and 18-22% for men, that's say 12-15 kilograms that needs to be deducted .

What we are left with is lean body weight, which is the total weight of your organs, bones, skin, muscles and blood. In this example 70-15= 55kg LBM.

You multiply this number by the minimum protein requirement which is 0.8g protein per KILOGRAM or 0.36g per Pound of goal body weight.
55 x 0.8g = 44g

That is the bare minimum that doesn't include the increased need for muscle repair or building with any exercise you may do.

If we factor this in, we will then raise the requirement to 1.0g per kilo or 0.42g per Pound.

55 x 1.0g = 55g

If you are doing cardio type training this will again be raised to around 1.2g/kg and 0.5g per pound of goal body weight.

55 x 1.2 = 66g

Endurance athletes are around 1.4g/kg, 55 x 1.4 = 77g

and intense strength trainers are around 2.0g/kg 55 x 2.0 =110g

Some web pages are misrepresenting the information either by accident or design stating 1g per pound of total body weight for the average person This is INSANE!! The average person is around 180 pounds (that's 180g protein they're being told to eat!!) This is simply too much and impossible for a post-op bariatric patient.

Now let's look at a couple of other things,

If you've had bariatric surgery, your absorption rate is approx. 20-30% lower than prior to surgery (reported average). So to combat this as a precaution you will need to eat 20-30% more protein . i.e. you minimum is 55g before surgery, after you'll need to add another 15g (approx.) and aim for 70g.

If you are menopausal, post menopausal or have had a hysterectomy. Your muscle mass declines with age, as muscle mass declines so does bone density, which can lead to osteoporosis. So, to help prevent bone density decline via muscle wastage, on average you'll need to eat about 5-10g more per day. 70+5-10 = 75- 80g

If you are eating low carb to lose weight, you can adjust your macros to work for you. This goes for everyone, bariatric or not.

Studies have shown that increasing your minimum protein intake by up to 30% can aid in weight loss and healthy outcomes, but anything over has no real benefit. So again, your minimum 55g + 30% = 70g (approx.)

Lets round this up and add a little frosting, 70-75g.

Or is you are a post menopausal bariatric 80g + 30% = 104g (approx.)
Or the average person at max intensity training 110g + 30% = 140g (approx.)

Obviously, the less body fat and more muscle you have, the higher your requirements will be, but no matter how you look at it, the average 70 kilogram /170 pound individual does not require 180g.

Eating too much protein can in fact have the opposite effect of the one desired as excess protein that can not be metabolized gets stored in the muscle as glycogen, and released from the muscles during gluconeogenesis to form glucose, so your max power efforts to avoid carbs by smashing the protein are in vain, as your body is making its own sugar, which creates an insulin response and as we know, insulin is our FAT STORAGE HORMONE !

So what do we take away from this?

What's a safe protein amount?

Be **smarter not harder** with your protein.

Aim for a baseline minimum intake of around 60.g for women and 65.g for men.

Then adjust this number to meet your specific post surgical and exercise needs.

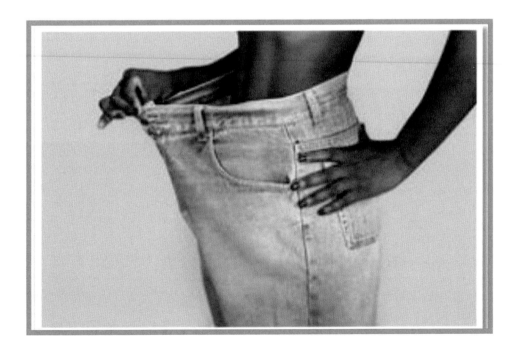

The Importance of Sleep

Sleep deficiency can increase your irritability, risk of depression and anxiety, decrease your learning ability, reaction time and problem solving; and even negatively impact your libido, and overall sense of wellbeing.

Sleep is an important factor when it comes to a well functioning metabolism and good weight loss results and the influence that diet has on sleep is just as important as the influence that sleep has on diet. Let me explain.

In a study published by The Journal of Clinical and Sleep Medicine, it was found that sleep was less restorative and more disrupted in those who ate an unbalanced diet high in saturated fat, sugar and low in dietary fibre. It found that fibre increased the instances of time spent in deep sleep, and conversely fats and sugars correlated with more time awake, more frequent arousals from sleep and less time spent in deep low wave sleep.

So, what we eat can influence the quality of our sleep, but on the other hand, the quality of our sleep can influence what we eat.

Sleep deprivation has the potential to change habitual feeding patterns due to its impact on the mechanisms that regulate hunger and satiety. Losing sleep can lead your body to down regulate metabolic processes to be less able to regulate blood sugar. This in turn leads to spikes in insulin an causes the body to process carbohydrate less efficiently and lose weight less effectively.

This is due to many factors, the most influential of which is hormone regulation.

Two hormones in particular are Ghrelin and Leptin. Ghrelin is responsible for triggering hunger, and Leptin is produced to stimulate feelings of satiety. When we lose sleep or get insufficient amounts of restorative sleep, these two hormones, (when disrupted by poor sleep), will trigger cravings, and contribute to improper eating habits as well as over eating.

Research by the University of Chicago found that dieters had better weight loss results when they slept more soundly and regularly achieved 7-8hrs of continuous sleep per night.

Sleep Hygiene

Sleep hygiene refers to the practices put into place to encourage regular patterns of restorative continuous sleep. (clean sleep practices). Some examples of Sleep Hygiene practices that you can employ are:

⇒ Take Magnesium. Magnesium effectively promotes sleep with its relaxing and calmative actions. A dose of 300mg 1hr-30 min prior to bed can alleviate the symptoms of insomnia and encourage a more restorative sleep. Go for Magnesium Malate as this is better absorbed.

⇒ Eat a balanced and healthy diet complete with wholefoods, fruits, vegetables and dietary fibre.

⇒ Set your bedtime to allow 8−8 1/2 hours in your bed, this should allow you enough time to actually get to sleep.

⇒ Last 30 min of the night to be technology free(computer /phone off). Technology i.e. playing on your smart phone, stimulates brain waves and disrupts your natural rhythms.

⇒ Remove caffeine and stimulants from your diet.

⇒ Use your bed for only two purposes, Sleep and (you know what the second one is). Make sure that this is your place to rest and recover.

⇒ Don't fight tiredness. Your body will have natural waves of tiredness that come and go, if you fight one wave, you will disrupt your rhythms and will find yourself 'wired' as a result.

⇒ Make sleep just as important as everything else you do. Remind yourself that part of your success relies on a healthy body-mind connection and sleep can help that process.

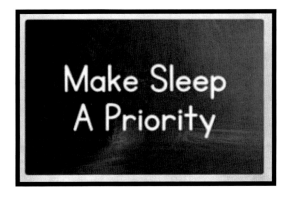
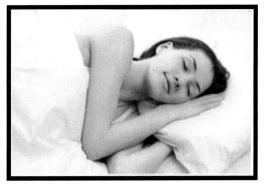

Fasting? Its ok 'once' in a while.

Whilst I do not recommend fasting as a rule and especially NOT to people with metabolic resistance and issues losing weight, a 'partial fasting' approach is included in some versions of this reset.

Fasting is thought to be and active thoughtful process of self-preservation in which life energy, otherwise used in digesting and utilising food, is concentrated on purifying and healing the body. For some it has a spiritual application, to others like myself, it is a methodical and scientific beginning to a new way of thinking.

How this applies to you is up to where your beliefs lie and dependant on what you want to get out of it.

What fasting may do for you:

- Take you mentally and physically away from the active process of eating, and give you space to recognise true hunger responses and your reactions and emotions associated with food and feeding. You are not going to be able to distract your feelings with food. You are going to address them and by using mindfulness techniques, put systems in place to heal your relationship with food.

- Free up energy otherwise used on actively digesting food, to cleanse the body of built up waste products, eliminate toxins and break addictive cycles as it helps to reduce our tolerance for harmful products.

Studies into fasting have reported positive results in lowering blood pressure, cholesterol, and oxidative stress. Also finding that insulin and inflammatory markers were also lowered in a clinically meaningful way. However, it most be noted that none of these studies were conducted on post-surgical weight loss patients with metabolic resistance.

Content provided in this book is of a general nature only and does not replace the information and advice provided by your own health care professionals. Always consult your own health providers for specific personal health and medical advice.

40

The scientific viewpoint

Things that occur in the body during fasting:

- Cellular Repair — New cells are created, old cells are broken down and dysfunctional proteins are removed from the cells.

- Insulin Decline — Insulin sensitivity improves, and lowered Insulin makes body fat more accessible for use.

- Human Growth Hormone (HGH) Increase: HGH is beneficial for weight loss and muscle growth.

- Norepinephrine Increase: (noradrenaline) is a fat burning hormone. *Changes in hormone levels during fasting may actually increase your metabolic rate.

How and why is it included in this Reset?

A partial 'fast' is included in the first couple of days of the Fresh Start Pouch Reset : Option # 1, to not only provide your body with the opportunity to simplify the processes and initiate proper hunger responses, but to also allow your mind to be cleared of your regular eating patterns, remove your daily triggers and start from scratch. A full day 'non-spiritual' fast is included in Option#2, to enhance this process by the removal of all temptations.

By removing your triggers and normal type meals, you are creating a clean slate to begin your new way of thinking and eating.

And a clean slate equals a FRESH START !

So are you Ready, Set…..RESET !

* Please note: Fasting for longer than the 24 hours set out in the Advanced Option of the Fresh Start Reset is not recommended nor supported. Fasting is not suitable for everyone, please check with your physician if you believe that you may have any conditions that could be negatively impacted by restriction of this type.

How to get a

Fresh Start,

Reset

and

Regain Control

Getting Ready

- **PREPARE YOUR MIND:** You want to remove distractions from the equation. So grab the calendar out, mark your days. Make sure that you start on a day when you are afforded the time to focus on you. OR, if you know that you work better on days where you are busy mentally, start on that day. It is about knowing yourself.

- **PREPARE YOUR EMOTIONAL RESPONSES:** If you know yourself , you know how you respond to stress situations. So get out your notebook and pen, and write down your fears, your reactions and strategies on how to overcome them. Keep your journal handy for your Reset homework.

- **PREPARE YOUR ENVIRONMENT:** Remove your triggers, clear your fridge, get rid of your bad snacks and treats. Take away the little temptations like the cookie barrel on the bench, even if it is empty. These are triggers to think about food. Tell your family and friends how they can support you through the next 2 weeks, tell them not to bring take out home, tell them to be gentle with you. Prepare them that you will be going through a transitional change and may be stressed out. Let the people on your support forum know that you are doing this and get their help. Check in daily.

- **PREPARE YOURSELF:** Don't begin unless you are well. Don't begin if you are full of anxiety. Don't begin unless you are ready.   Preparing yourself also means preparing yourself for success, and this includes being confident in your plan and your goals.

Most of all , before you go forward into this new journey, stop. Take stock of how far you have come, where your were this time last year, or the year before. Think about where you came from. You might be struggling right now, but the progress you have made so far is nothing short of amazing. Congratulate yourself, and be sure to congratulate others.

" I am worthy

of

100% of my effort,

100% of my time

&

100% of my Love"

PICK YOUR RESET

1. **Beginners:** For those of you who want a gentle introduction into reset without 'too much' restriction or if you feel like your portions are in check but need to work on some food relationships and triggers . **PAGE: 49**

2. **Intermediate (Original):** The 'Original Reset' , Transitional, thoughtful. The beginning will bring you back to basics to cleanse your body, encourage healing, calm your system and decrease inflammation. Aiming to clear mental, emotional and physical pathways and put you in touch with your true relationship with food and feeding. Slowing things down, removing obstacles and nourishing your mind and body. You will be reintroduced to your satiety point with mindful eating practices. You'll take notice of your signals and identify strategies to manage cravings. Transitioning to more frequent eating and establish snack routines to aid in delivering your protein and nutrient requirements using appropriate portion control, and prepare yourself to move forward into your ongoing weight loss or lifestyle eating plan. **PAGE: 53**

3. **Advanced (Fasting Start):** Takes you on the same journey with food, however begins with a full day of therapeutic, non-spiritual fasting. Your meal options are the same, your instructions are the same, except you will start with an aim to focus and allow your body to begin from a different mindset, the only thing different are the days when you transition. **PAGE: 91**

4. **Vegan/Vegetarian Reset:** This version allows for differences in dietary design whilst ensuring that nutrition needs are met during the reset. Less restrictive but may challenge your true refined carb-addict. **PAGE: 97**

5. **Hypo-Glycaemia/Diabetic Support Reset:** Designed to maintain balanced insulin/glucose levels and minimise the impact of rapid drops in blood sugar. This option would be a more gentle transition into the world of low-carb and ketogenic diet planning. **PAGE: 107**

6. **Exercise/Workout Support Reset:** If you just cannot lay down the weights for a few days for the initial stages of reset and want a plan that is going to support your energy needs while getting you back on track. **PAGE: 115**

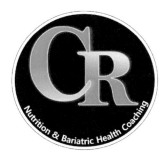

Fresh Start

Beginners

Reset

Beginners Reset Rules

Follow ALL Original Reset days except for the variations below.

Days 1 and 2

Follow all specifications:

However you can add your choice of:

- 2 x low-carb protein shakes (Breakfast & Lunch)

(OR)

- 1 x low- carb Protein Shake (Breakfast) and 1 x Green Apple (lunch)

(OR)

- 1 x Apple (lunch) and 1 cup Cooked Broccoli with Bone Broth (dinner)

Days 3 to 5

Follow all specifications:

However you can add your choice of:

- 1 x low-carb protein shake (Breakfast or Lunch)

(OR)

- 1 x Green Apple (lunch)

(OR)

- 1 cup Cooked Broccoli with Bone Broth (alternate to the main meal)

Days 6 to 9

Follow all specifications:

However you can add your choice of:

1 x low-carb protein shake **(OR)** 1 x Green Apple for Breakfast.

Days 10 to 14

FOLLOW ORIGINAL RESET INSTRUCTION 100%

"I will make decisions without worrying about what others may think."

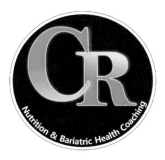

Fresh Start

Original Reset

Original Reset Days 1 and 2

Begin the day with:

- 1-2 tsp of apple cider vinegar (ACV)– with the 'Mother' in ½ cup of water. (ACV)

  Apple Cider Vinegar has many healthful properties. Its nutritional value is emphasised by active enzymes and good bacteria, and acetic acid helps lower blood pressure. It aids in digestive function and helps boost immunity. If ACV is not to your taste, you can substitute for another probiotic beverage such as 1/4 cup of Milk Kefir, water Kefir or Kombucha.

Throughout the day:

- Drink at a limit of 1 cup every half hour, of the following nourishing fluids but **limit to 10 cups** per day:

  - **Bone broth** — bone broth is recommended as it contains many essential nutrients and electrolytes, as well as containing approximately 5g of protein per cup.
  - Chicken, beef and vegetable broths.
  - Cabbage soup broth.

You may dink **unlimited water**, with the aim to consume up to 64oz/2 litres in a day. (This is total volume of all liquids)

You may have 2 cups of caffeinated beverages. Recommended in the first half of the day. These must **NOT contain dairy,** to be consumed BLACK.

You may drink the following herbal teas in unlimited quantities;

- Lemon Balm, Green tea , Peppermint or Dandelion
- Other — no sugar or no-fruit added herbal teas.
  - ⇒ Feel free to add cinnamon, turmeric or ginger for blood sugar regulation and anti-inflammatory action.
  - ⇒ If you simply cannot do plain water, you can infuse water with slices of fruit or vegetables.

Other:

- ⇒ **Stay away** from sugar free popsicles and Gatorade type drinks as these give the sensation of sugar ingestion, and can trigger insulin spikes in some individuals.
- ⇒ Continue with your supplement routine.
- ⇒ If you get a headache, tale your normal headache pain relief.
- ⇒ Try and rest as much as you can.
- ⇒ Journal or post about your struggles and successes.
- ⇒ Take your probiotic prior to bed so that it has time to properly colonise your GI tract.

Reset Self Assessment Homework Day 1

You will do a series of writing tasks as part of your journey. They are for you, so be honest with yourself. Answer the following:	
What eating actions lead you to surgery? (Overeating, take out every night etc.)	
What eating actions lead you to reset? (Overeating, take out every night etc.)	
What does food 'mean' to you? (comfort, pleasure, fuel etc.)	
Why do you indulge? **What are your triggers?**	
How do you feel when you indulge?	

Write down your 3 main food triggers and strategies to overcome these.	
Trigger:	Strategy:
Trigger:	Strategy:
Strategy:	Strategy:

What is going to work for you?

Will taking 10 x long deep breaths work? Drinking a glass of water, or splashing your face ?

Take notice of your environment and the tools you have and come up with ways to diffuse cravings.

TASK: When craving hits, get up from your position and take a walk. In the office? Get up, get a glass of water or go to the restroom. At home? Go outside or into another room. With every step think.

"This is just a feeling and it will pass". Walk off the craving. If it comes back, repeat the process.

"*I am in control of what and when I eat..
And I have the strength to STOP comfort eating.*"

Reset Self Assessment Homework Day 2

You will do a series of writing tasks as part of your journey. **They are for you, so be honest with yourself. Answer the following:**	
What eating actions lead you to surgery? **(Overeating, take out every night etc.)**	
What eating actions lead you to reset? **(Overeating, take out every night etc.)**	
What does food 'mean' to you? **(comfort, pleasure, fuel etc.)**	
Why do you indulge? **What are your triggers?**	
How do you feel when you indulge?	

Write down your 3 main food triggers and strategies to overcome these.	
Trigger:	**Strategy:**
Trigger:	**Strategy:**
Strategy:	**Strategy:**

TASK: Lay in a darkened room with your eyes closed and start to count back from 1000, as you do this breathe in deeply and out slowly. With every breath release the negative emotion you feel about your weight, your body and food. With every breath in think "I will succeed".

*"I am in full control of
my impulses... I can
find more productive
ways of comforting
myself
other than eating."*

BONE BROTH

* You can get bones by simply asking your butcher.

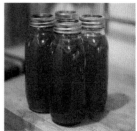

- Start with good quality bones/ chicken frames. Preferably organic and hormone-free .

- Add 1/4 –1/2 cup vinegar (depending on how large the batch you're making).

- Add any vegetables you want to add, and water to cover. Because of their extremely high nutritional content, be sure to add some dark leafy greens to the mix.

- Let this sit for 30 minutes to an hour, (this allows the vinegar to leech vital nutrients out of the bones). Bring to a boil and remove any scum that appears on the surface.

- Continue to simmer anywhere from 4-24 hours, the longer the simmer, the more nutrients will be drawn out of the bones.

- When done, you can measure your 1 Cup serving size into mason jars , and store in the fridge for when you need them.

- A layer of fat will form on the top of each jar and solidify when cool, Do not remove this as the fat has many vital nutrients and will aid in promoting satiety.

  To make a vegetable broth: Make the same way, simply omit the bones.

HERBAL TEA

For a cool refreshing drink, why not make iced tea.

- Steep 4-6 bags/ serves of your favourite herbal tea, in 2 cups of boiling water and let sit for 1-2 hours.

- When cool, mix with 4 cups cold water, and 1 –2 tablespoons of Lemon or Lime juice. (you may like to slice the lemons and/or a 1inch piece of ginger sliced finely; and steep them in the boiling water for a zesty treat)

Iced Green tea with lemon and ginger is refreshing and cleansing.

The benefits of...
Bone Broth

Bone broth is a powerhouse of nutrients and minerals. It includes immune system supporting and healing compounds such as collagen and amino acids such as glutamine, glycine and proline. These compounds work synergistically to help heal the gut lining which in turn increases nutrient absorption of other essential vitamins and minerals from your diet.

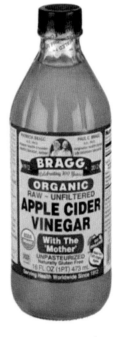

A single cup of bone broth has around 5g of protein and provides essential electrolytes needed to ward off the effects of ketogenic transition (i.e. Keto flu).

Whilst it is an acquired taste for some, you can customize your broth by adding lemongrass, ginger, a touch of fish sauce and chili and turn it into a healthy Pho' alternative, or add any spices you prefer to make it your own.

Apple Cider Vinegar

Apple cider vinegar is high in acetic acid which has been shown to lower blood glucose and improve insulin sensitivity major benefit to those with diabetes. It is a powerful antioxidant, antibiotic and antifungal.

There have been several studies that have shown that Apple Cider Vinegar can make you feel fuller for longer and it has an impact on satiety; which in turn is of benefit for weight loss. The consumption of apple cider vinegar can help reduce triglyceride levels, and therefore reduce risk factors associated with heart disease. It is also a helpful aid for denaturing proteins in the gut and therefore a digestive aid.

The best kind of Apple Cider vinegar is the liquid variety that contains 'the mother', strains of live culture bacteria which a reportedly responsible for many of the gut health associations. Whilst ACV is available in pill form, a 2005 study found that the actual content of the capsules was debatable, and another anecdotal report had woman receive oesophageal burns due to a capsule getting stuck in her throat after swallowing.

So include ACV liquid if you can tolerate it, if not, why not try Kombucha or Kefir.

What is Kombucha

Kombucha is a probiotic beverage that is made by fermenting tea. It has a natural effervescence (fizz) and as well as the probiotics, it also contains antioxidants, B vitamins and is widely used for its many health benefits inclusive of promoting a healthy immune system and preventing constipation.

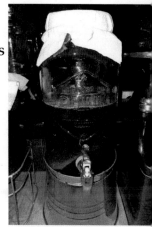

Kombucha allegedly originated in Asia, and can be linked back as early as 220BCE with reported records of it being used in Russia and Eastern Europe. So it has been around for quite some time, and once again we are becoming aware of its benefits. Sweet brewed black tea is used to feed the SCOBY which in turn ferments the tea into the beverage. This is sometimes referred to as "Kombucha mushroom tea", but Kombucha is not a mushroom, it is a SCOBY — which stands for "Symbiotic-Colony/Culture — Of –Bacteria and Yeast".

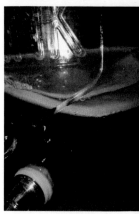

The billions of individual bacterium and yeast gather and join together to form a colony. Working as one to feed on the sugar in the tea, growing bigger until they become the SCOBY. These SCOBY's form on the surface of your tea and take on the appearance of milky coloured wet jelly-fish-like pancake (Sounds appealing doesn't it!!) But it is nature doing its magical thing!

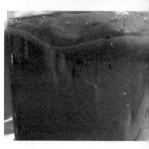

Top: Kombucha brew tank; **Middle:** multi layer scoby growth—mature scoby . **Bottom:** Yeast filament strands. This is what a normal healthy scoby looks like as it ferments your Kombucha.

What benefits are there in drinking Kombucha?

As already stated, Kombucha contains probiotics and beneficial yeasts, which promote healthy gut flora which is linked with more efficient immune response as well as enhanced metabolic function and better digestion. Kombucha can help ease the onset and occurrence of constipation and also help detoxify the body. Kombucha is not a 'cure-all' but what it is, is a 'balancer', it helps bring the body back into balance so that it can heal itself.

It is a lot gentler on the taste buds than apple cider vinegar but still has a vinegar like taste, as most fermented products do.

How do you make Kombucha

It is actually quite simple, and only differs on how you want to begin

1. Make a strong black tea (the quantity depends on the size jar you are using– for this example lets say 8 cups/ 2 litres, therefore use around 10 tea bags)

2. Add approx. 1/2 cup – 3/4 cup of sugar per 2 litres.

3. Sterilize a container – you do this with hot water and distilled vinegar only.

4. If you are lucky enough to obtain or be gifted with a Scoby, you can add this to your cooled sweet black tea. Or alternatively add a fresh bottle of Kombucha with live cultures. (you are looking for UNFLAVOURED, raw, organic and live)

5. Cover the mouth of the jar with cheese cloth or kitchen towel and affix with rubber bands. Let ferment anywhere between 7 and 30 days (weather dependant), begin tasting after approx. 5 days. Your Kombucha should be more tart than sweet and mildly acidic (vinegar-like).

6. When it has fermented to your taste, you can bottle it in smaller jars, and also introduce a secondary ferment cycle by adding a few berries , ginger or fruit pieces , to flavour it further. (second ferment is not necessary)

- Do not use fruit tea or flavoured tea as this can taint or kill your Scoby, as well as induce a perfume like taste to the brew.

- Be careful with surface spray, antibacterial spray or insect sprays, as your scobys can absorb these from the air and will result in a tainted brew or dead scoby.

What are the nutritional benefits?

Kombucha is great source of probiotics (healthy bacteria) and beneficial for the gastrointestinal tract,. It contains many beneficial strains of bacteria that can aid in digestive function, boot immunity, enhance nutrient absorption and rebalance natural gut bacteria leading to higher levels of well being.

Its made using sugar, should I be avoiding it?

Whilst sugar is used in the production of Kombucha, the sugar content of the drink is actually quite low. This is because the sugar is used to feed the yeast and bacteria of the scoby which in turn ferments the drink. So , by the end, the majority of the sugar will have been consumed by the bacteria.

Does Kombucha contain alcohol or caffeine?

There is a regular amount of caffeine that you would have in a cup of tea or coffee and small amounts of alcohol due the fermenting of the sugars. The more sugar added the more alcoholic it will be – which is not the aim, but rather a warning. You can always make your Kombucha with 1/2 as much sugar to begin with and sweeten with stevia prior to drinking.

What is Kefir

Milk Kefir is fermented sour dairy, with a consistency and taste similar to thin yogurt. Due to the fermentation of the lactose in the milk. Kefir Grains look like small cauliflower florets, these are in fact Scoby's (like Kombucha) and can grow to the size of walnuts , but generally multiply into smaller 'grain –like colonies. The taste, texture, and bacteria strains of the Kefir are dependent on the type of milk that is fermented, however the same facts rings true for all, the grains break down and eat the milk sugars (lactose) , supplying you with a *mostly* lactose free yoghurt-like drink. Kefir is found to be very tolerable to those with lactose intolerances. Fermented dairy products also have a slower transit time in the digestive tract, and therefore can reduce the instance of dairy related dumping syndrome, as seen in many after weight loss surgery.

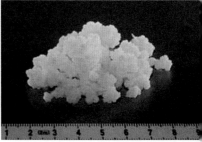

Milk Kefir Grains

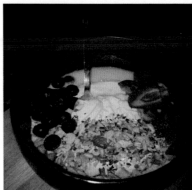

There are varieties of Kefir that thrive in various other liquids, and again their composition and benefits vary from type to type. Water kefir is grown for up to a few days at room   temperature in water with sugar, and often dried fruit like figs or apricots.

Kefir Yoghurt Breakfast Bowl: After fermentation, let kefir drip through cheesecloth to remove the whey. The end product a thick Greek style yoghurt. The whey can then be used to ferment vegetable or be added as a protein source to smoothies or cooking.

Kefir contains several important strains beneficial bacteria not commonly found in yogurt, *Lactobacillus Caucasus, Leuconostoc, Acetobacter species, and Streptococcus species.* As well as beneficial yeasts, which control and eliminate harmful yeasts in the body. Kefir is a great source of:

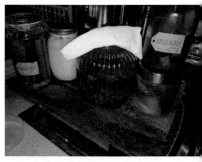

- Tryptophan—which is a precursor to serotonin and there fore important for mental health.

Vegetables fermenting in whey.

- B12—crucial for DNA, nerve and blood a healthy brain and immune system.

- Calcium—cardiovascular health and bone density.

- Magnesium - is important for over 300 biological   processes in the body.

- Biotin— cardiovascular, nerve and metabolic functions.

- Vitamin K—Bone health, cardiovascular health and blood clotting.

To make kefir, add grains to milk and let ferment over night (weather dependent).

Days 3 –5

Begin the day with:
- With your ACV, Kombucha or kefir.
- Remember to take your supplements

Throughout the day:
- You may drink <u>no more</u> than **4 cups** per day of the following:
    - Clear beef, chicken or vegetable broth.
      Can now include up to **3 tbsp** of **small pieces** of meat and vegetable but NO STARCHY VEGETABLES
    - Bone broth.
    - Cabbage soup broth.
- You may dink **unlimited water,** with the aim to consume up to 64oz/2 litres in a day.
- You may have 2 cups of caffeinated beverages. These must **NOT contain dairy,** to be consumed BLACK.
- You may continue to drink herbal teas in Unlimited quantities;
    ⇒ Still S**tay away** from sugary tasting products/drinks

You will be including to your day ONE MEAL

This ONE meal can be had at either breakfast, lunch OR dinner. That choice is yours.
- 2- 3oz (80-100g) of chicken or fish, grilled ,poached or roasted;
- 1/4 -1/2 cup of low carb or low GI vegetables (see list)
    - Broccoli, Green beans, Spinach or Brussel Sprouts etc.
- You may add butter, salt and pepper to your vegetables and or Olive Oil + Apple Cider vinegar dressing.

For Gastric Bypass/ Duodenal Switch
⇒ **Try NOT to physically eat more than** 3/4 cup of food per meal.

For sleeve and Band
⇒ **Try NOT to physically eat more than** 1 cup of food per meal.

Other:
⇒ Continue with your supplement routine.
⇒ Journal or post about your struggles and successes.
⇒ Take your probiotic prior to bed so that it has time to properly colonise your GI tract.
⇒ REMEMBER NOT TO DRINK WITH YOUR MEAL. Do not drink fluids at least 15 min prior and A MINIMUM of 30 minutes after eating solid foods. (does not apply to soup with pieces in it)

Reset Self Assessment Homework Day 3

Think about your day:	
What challenges did you experience?	
Is there a way to deter this in the future?	
Think about your first solid meal:	
How did it make you feel to prepare the meal?	
What was it like taking that first bite? Did you encounter any feelings or emotions?	
At what point did you start feeling full?	

FIRST MEAL INSTRUCTIONS

Serve yourself a 2-3oz/80-100g piece of chicken of fish on a normal size dinner plate. Next to that , put 3-4 green beans and 2 small broccoli florets, add your dressing and before you dig in, take a photo and a mental picture of the size of your meal. Realise that **YOU HAVE A TINY STOMACH**

Take small meaningful bites and chew slowly.

Put your knife and fork down between bites and allow the food to go down. Take notice of the food and how it feels in your stomach before taking the next bite. STOP when you begin to feel pressure, This is your stomach stretching to accommodate. **If you feel this... STOP. YOU ARE DONE.**

It takes approximately 10-15 minutes for your stomach and brain to make the connection that you are full.

PUT THE FORK DOWN! And WAIT.

At the 30 minute mark, if you find that you are still hungry, then finish your meal, or have a cup of broth. BUT ONLY IF YOU ARE TRULY HUNGRY — don't cheat yourself by not being honest.

Repeat the process for the next two days.

*"I will develop
an
intuition
for
when I am full."*

Reset Self Assessment Homework Day 4

Think about your day:	
What challenges did you experience?	
Is there a way to deter this in the future?	
Think about your Second solid meal:	
How did it make you feel to prepare the meal?	
What was it like taking that first bite? Did you encounter any feelings or emotions?	
At what point did you start feeling full?	
What was different from yesterday?	
What have you discovered?	

Task: Go back to your realistic goal setting.

Read over your goals, and thinking about your last few days ask yourself…

- Are your goals still realistic?
- How do you feel about them?
- Do they need to be modified?

*"I have self discipline
and can easily resist
the temptation
of unhealthy food."*

Reset Self Assessment Homework Day 5

Think about your day:	
What challenges did you experience?	
Is there a way to deter this in the future?	
Think about your Third solid meal	
How did it make you feel to prepare the meal?	
What was it like taking that first bite? Did you encounter any feelings or emotions?	
At what point did you start feeling full?	
What was different from yesterday?	
What have you discovered?	

Task: Go back to your self connection examples.

Read over how you describe yourself, and thinking about your last few days ask yourself...

- Is there anything I can add to this list?
- What has challenging my associations with food shown me about myself?
- Are any of your original self perceptions challenged?

"I listen to my body and easily know when I am truly hungry."

GET FAMILIAR WITH
PORTION SIZES

A **4 oz.** piece of chicken is approximately the same size as a deck of cards. Your piece of protein should **be roughly this size.**

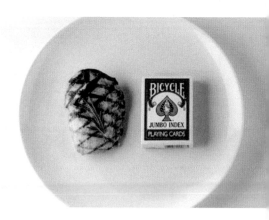

CHOOSE LOW CARB VEGETABLES TO ACCOMPANY YOUR PROTEIN

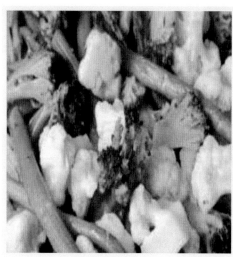

You can steam, boil or sauté 1/2 to 1 cup (follow the Surgery specific recommendation) of the following vegetables.

- Broccoli
- Green Beans
- Cauliflower
- Asparagus
- Spinach
- Zucchini

* Mushrooms
* Broccoli rabe
* Cabbage
* Kale
* Brussel Sprouts
* Asian Greens

ADD SOME FATS

- Sauté in olive oil
- Add a little butter to your vegetables
- Make vinaigrette dressing with a touch of olive oil, some apple cider vinegar , a squeeze of lemon , salt and Pepper.
- Use it to dress up your meal.

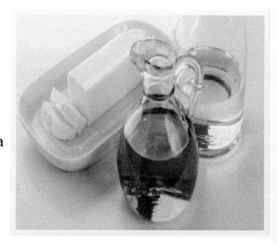

Low carb Foods

MEAT AND SEAFOOD

- Beef
- Veal
- Lamb
- Pork
- Fowl (turkey, chicken, duck, goose, hen, quail)
- Organ Meats
- Game Meats
- Exotic Meats (such as ostrich and emu)
- Cod
- Flounder
- Sole
- Haddock
- Halibut
- Sardine
- Swordfish
- Tuna
- Trout
- Salmon
- Catfish
- Bass
- Crab
- Shrimp
- Lobster
- Squid

LOW CARB SEASONING

- Salt and Pepper
- Vinegar
- Ground Cinnamon
- Most Hot Sauces
- Pre-mixed Seasonings (check labels)
- Yellow Mustard
- Dill
- Chives, Basil, Oregano, Rosemary, Thyme, etc.

OILS AND FATS

- Olive oil
- Coconut oil
- Grass-fed butter
- Walnut Oil
- MCT oil
- Avocado oil
- Fish oil

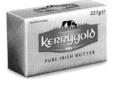

LOW CARB FRUIT AND V

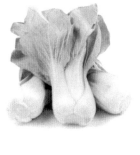

·1/2 cup serve:

- Spinach
- Parsley
- Avocado
- Radish
- Lettuce
- Bok Choy
- Celery

1/4 cup Serve

- Mushrooms
- Garlic (1/2 clove)
- Pokeberry Shoots
- Cabbage
- Asparagus (3 pieces)
- Yellow Squash
- Raspberries
- Cauliflower
- Broccoli
- Cucumber

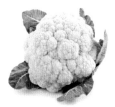

ALSO EAT

- Eggs
- Cheese (check carbs on label as some cheeses can have higher carbs than others)
- Heavy Cream
- Nuts and Seeds (in moderation)
- Stevia for sweeteners
- Zero-carb protein waters
- Low carb (under 8g per serve) protein shakes
- Dill pickles
- Sugar free pudding and gelatine

REMEMBER

- Drink Water
- Eat a variety of wholefoods
- Limit saturated fats
- Don't exceed your protein or carb limits
- Don't exceed calories
- Balance you gut
- Get moving.

Days 6 to 9

Begin the day with:
- With your ACV, Kombucha or kefir.
- Remember to take your supplements

Throughout the day:

Water is unlimited but you MUST now be consuming a minimum 64oz/2 litre in a day.

You may drink **no more** than **2 cups** per day of your broth/soup type fluids:

⇒ You MUST ensure adequate hydration to help the liver and kidneys eliminate toxins from your body.

⇒ You may have 2 cups of caffeinated beverages. You can now add 1 Tbsp. of heavy whipping cream.

⇒ You can drink herbal teas in unlimited quantities;

⇒ Continue to **stay away** from sugary tasting products.

Your Meals:

You will be adding more to your diet in the next 3 days.

Its time to add some snacks.

In **addition to** your 2-3oz. Chicken/fish and Vegetable meal, at whatever time you choose, you can now add 2 from the following (or suggestions on next page) to have as a mid-morning and mid-afternoon snack;

- Half a boiled egg in a lettuce leaf with ¼ avocado + 1 tsp of real egg mayo

- 10 almonds (or) 10 pistachios and 4 Strawberries.

- 6 slices of cucumber with cream cheese/cottage cheese or feta (1 tsp on each) and 2 slices of ham divided into 6.

CHEW SLOWLY AND MINDFULLY DURING ALL MEALS

- 10 green beans with a tbsp. of Persian feta or chopped dill pickle mixed with cream cheese

- 1 oz. of chicken or turkey breast with 4-6 cheddar cheese cubes.

- ¼ cup blueberries and 10 almonds or pistachios

- 2 roll ups – e.g. salami/pepperoni wrapped around any deli cheese like mozzarella, provolone, cheddar

- 2 bacon wrapped asparagus spears.

Other:

⇒ Continue with your supplement routine.

⇒ Journal or post about your struggles and successes.

⇒ Take your probiotic prior to bed so that it has time to properly colonise your GI tract.

⇒ REMEMBER NOT TO DRINK WITH YOUR MEAL. Do not drink fluids at least 15 min prior and A MINIMUM of 30 minutes after eating solid foods.

RESET SNACK IDEAS

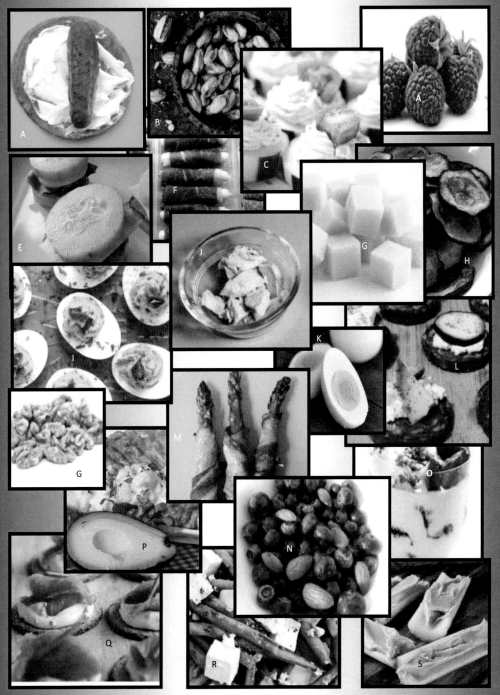

RESET SNACK IDEAS: A. Ham cream cheese + dill pickle roll up **B.**15 pistachios **C.**6 slices cucumber + 1 tbsp. cream cheese + 3 cherry tomatoes halved **D.**1/4 cup raspberries **E.**6 slices of cucumber + 1 oz. cheddar (or 1 tbsp. cream cheese) and 1 oz. ham **F.** Mozzarella stick salami roll up **G.** 1 oz. Cheese + 1 oz. nuts **H.** Zucchini chips (equivalent 1/2 a zucchini) **I.** Avocado devilled egg **J.** 1 oz. chicken **K.**1 boiled egg **L.**4 pieces of salami with cucumber and cottage cheese **M.** 2-3 bacon wrapped asparagus spears **N.** 1/4 cup blueberries + 10 almonds **O.** 60g Kefir or Greek yoghurt + 2 strawberries + 1/2 tbsp. nuts **P.** boiled egg and avocado salad lettuce cup **Q.** 4 whole wheat crackers + smoked salmon + 1 tbsp. cream cheese **R.** 10 green beans + 1 oz. feta **S.** 2 sticks of celery + 1 tbsp. Nut

Reset Self Assessment Homework Day 6

Thinking about your day...	
What triggers were experienced?	
What strategies did you use to make the right choices?	
What could have been done differently?	
Did you listen to your stomach or did you let emotions control actions ?	
When I wait between bites, I can feel...?	
Do I know when to stop? Do I stop?	

Things to ask yourself

- Did I get my 64oz/2 litres of water?
- Did I chew slowly and mindfully?
- Did I recognise my 'satiety point'? And did I acknowledge it or ignore it?
- Did I take all my supplements?
- Did I manage my temptations?
- Am I dedicated?
- Am I prepared for tomorrow?

"I will restrain myself from eating too much."

Reset Self Assessment Homework Day 7

Thinking about your day...	
What triggers were experienced?	
What strategies did you use to make the right choices?	
What could have been done differently?	
Did you listen to your stomach or did you let emotions control actions ?	
What have I discovered about myself?	
How in 'control' am I feeling?	
After one week on the program I am feeling?	
Tomorrow will be?	

"*My hunger naturally subsides*

after I've eaten enough."

Reset Self Assessment Homework Day 8

Thinking about your day...	
What triggers were experienced?	
What strategies did you use to make the right choices?	
What could have been done differently?	
Did you listen to your stomach or did you let emotions control actions ?	
During this process I have struggled with?	
During this process I have overcome?	
During this process I have been surprised by my ability to?	
At Day 8 I am feeling.....	

*" My mind has
a strong and healthy
connection
to my body."*

Reset Self Assessment Homework Day 9

Thinking about your day...	
What triggers were experienced?	
What strategies did you use to make the right choices?	
What could have been done differently?	
Did you listen to your stomach or did you let emotions control actions ?	
When I think about my progress I feel?	
Knowing that I get to eat a full day of meals from now on makes me feel….	
I feel like I will face challenges of…..	
Strategies I will use to overcome these challenges will be….	

"I am transforming into someone who is naturally motivated to eat healthy."

SNACKS

Blueberries are a great source of antioxidants. They boost mental function, aid digestion, promote heart health, are beneficial for our skin and aid in weight loss. Limit your serve to 1/4 cup.

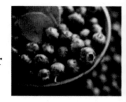

Almonds contain healthy fats, vitamin E, protein, magnesium and fibre. Almonds can help lower blood sugar levels, lower blood pressure and even help to reduce cholesterol. 10 nuts with some berries would be an adequate mid-morning snack.

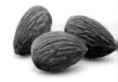

Cheese is a great source of calcium, which is one of the most lacking nutrients in the standard western diet. Cheese also contains protein, phosphorus, zinc, vitamin A and vitamin B12. Don't go overboard on the cheese though, it is still high in calories. A 1 oz. piece with some nuts or meat should help to satisfy your 'snacketite'.

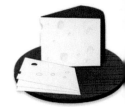

Meats like chicken breast or tinned fish are a perfect option to take to work. You can use cold cuts of meat like ham, salami or provolone to roll up into mini 'wraps'. Fill them with cream cheese and a pickle for a crunchy protein filled afternoon snack.

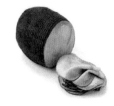

Avocados are nutrient rich and a great source of vitamins C, E, K, and B-6, as well as riboflavin, niacin, folate, pantothenic acid, magnesium, and potassium. They also provide lutein, betacarotene, as well as omega-3 fatty acids. While on reset, keep your serve to 1/4 avocado per snack or meal.

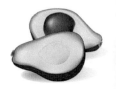

Eggs are a great source of high quality protein. Eggs also contain selenium, vitamin D, B6, B12 and minerals such as zinc, iron and copper. More than 50% of the protein found in eggs is in the whites.

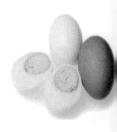

"Having confidence in myself is becoming easier with each passing day."

Days 10 to 14

Begin the day with:
- With your ACV, Kombucha or kefir.
- Remember to take your supplements

Throughout the day:

Water is unlimited but you MUST now be consuming a minimum 64oz/2 litre in a day.

You no longer need to have soup, unless you want it.

You may have 2 cups of caffeinated beverages.

- You can now add **1 tbsp. of heavy whipping cream**, and may add **a NO CARB sweetener** if you wish such as Xylitol, Stevia or Splenda.
- You may continue to drink herbal tea.

Your Meals:

The next four days are about transition.

You will have more choices:

- You will have your **ONE** meal of protein and vegetable as you have each day, but from today onwards you can choose 2-3 oz. of **any dense protein** source i.e. beef, lamb, pork etc
- You will incorporate **TWO** snacks into your day that contain either a fat, a protein or Both.

CHEW SLOWLY AND

MINDFULLY DURING

ALL MEALS

Like those in the list supplied for days 6 to 9.

You will also incorporate **TWO SMALL** protein and fat containing meals for Breakfast and Lunch; Some examples include;

- A 1-Egg, bacon and cheese mini quiche
- Salmon/tuna salad (1 cup leafy salad)
- Lettuce roll up wraps – filling with ham, cream cheese, a couple slices of capsicum and scallions etc.
- 1-2 oz. of protein (meat or Tofu) with 1 cup of salad greens and feta cheese oil dressing or ½ cup veg.
- Boiled egg and green beans
- 1 -2 oz. of chicken or salmon with ¼ avocado and tsp of aioli.

Other:
⇒ Continue with your supplement routine.
⇒ Journal or post about your struggles and successes.
⇒ Take your probiotic prior to bed so that it has time to properly colonise your GI tract.
⇒ REMEMBER NOT TO DRINK WITH YOUR MEAL. Do not drink fluids at least 15 min prior and A MINIMUM of 30 minutes after eating solid foods.

Reset Self Assessment Homework Day 10-14

Thinking about your last days...	
What were your biggest challenges?	
What do you need to remain mindful of?	
What were your biggest successes or revelations?	
Do you feel that you are in better control now over negative food associations?	
Are your intakes at your meals smaller than before or have you been pushing it?	
Have you used your time effectively to set up strategies that WORK at keeping you on track?	
Have you done your best to use mindfulness to control your relationship with food?	
Are you ready to move forward into the CR Nutrition Balanced Macros Plan © to keep your success going?	

Tasks for transition:

- Get yourself your **Balanced Macros Program – The Complete Solution to Bariatric Keto** and your personalized macronutrient profile report so you can transition smoothly and stock your pantry.

- Make sure you connect with your support group friends and peers, they are an excellent source of guidance and can help you with your meal planning ideas.

- Make sure you have downloaded a meal tracker application like My Fitness Pal, you'll need to track your intake after resetting until you know what you can do.

- Continue your supplement and probiotic routine.

"I am transforming into someone who lives a healthy and balanced life."

SMALL MEAL IDEAS

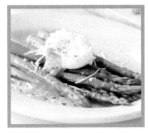

- **Butter and Garlic sautéed asparagus with poached egg and parmesan cheese.** It is as easy and as straight forward as it sounds. Cook asparagus and top with egg and parmesan.

- **Grilled bacon wrapped cheesy asparagus.** Sauté asparagus until tender, remove from heat. Lay out 3 pieces of bacon and lay 2 asparagus spear on each. Add a sprinkle of grated cheddar and par-mesan cheese, rollup and place back in frypan until bacon is crisp.

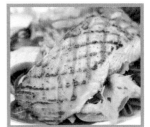

- **Grilled salmon and avocado salad.** 1/2 cup of green salad leaves, 2oz. of grilled salmon, 1/4 avocado sliced. Dress with a vinaigrette made of 1 Tbsp. Apple cider vinegar, 1 Tbsp. Olive oil, 1 tsp. Lemon juice, salt and pepper.

- **Avocado Devilled Eggs.** Boil 4-6 medium sized eggs. Allow to cool and then peel. Slice eggs in half and gently remove the yolks , emptying into a bowl. Add to the yolks, 1/2 an Avocado, 1 Tbsp. white vinegar, 1 tsp curry powder, salt and pepper, 1 tsp lemon juice and mix until smooth. Using a spoon or piping bag, refill the hollows with the mix. Place the halves in a container with a lid and store in the refrigerator. Eat 2 halves for your snack, or together with some green salad leaves for your meal.

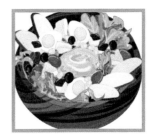

- **Salads.** You can't seem to go wrong with salad and you are only limited by your imagination . You can try chicken and Persian feta on baby spin-ach with radish. Or make a Caesar salad (without croutons). Try a warm Thai beef salad, exchanging noodles for thin zucchini ribbons, use fresh mint, cilantro/coriander and parsley together with baby spinach and dressed with sesame oil , chili and fish sauce.

REMEMBER:

- Small meals contain 1 1/2 –2 oz. of dense protein
- Where as your **main meal** contains 2-3 oz. (no more) of dense protein.
  (unless otherwise specified)
- Refer to your low-carb food list for your options.

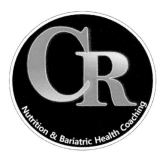

Fresh Start

Advanced

Reset

Fasting Start Advanced Reset

DAY	INSTRUCTION "HOW TO EAT"	SELF-ASSESSMENT "What Homework task?"
1	Follow **Fasting Start Advanced Reset.** **First Day Instructions**	Follow **Original Reset Homework :** Days 1
2 and 3	Follow **Original Reset Instructions** : Days 1-2	Follow **Original Reset Homework :** Days 2-3
4 to 7	Follow **Original Reset Instructions** : Days 3-5 (on all 4 days)	Follow **Original Reset Homework :** Days 4, 5, 6 and 7
8 to 11	Follow **Original Reset Instructions** : Days 6-9 (on all 4 days)	Follow **Original Reset Homework :** Days 8, 9, 10 and 11
12 to 14	Follow **Original Reset Instructions** : Days 10-14 (on all 3 days)	Follow **Original Reset Homework :** Days 12 to 14

Good luck on your journey, we will see you at the finish line.

Day 1

Full Day Fast

The Fresh Start—Fasting Start Reset, gives you the option to start your 14 days off with a clear head and an empty stomach.

Some people find the fasting hard, and it can be mentally challenging, so be prepared by scheduling your day one on a day where you will be able to ignore the calls to eat and ignore the temptations. Schedule your first day to begin on day that you can dedicate to you, to rest, to focus and to reflect.

How to begin Day one

- Upon waking you will have 1 cup of hot water with 2 tsp of ACV and 1 tsp of lemon or lime juice.

- You may have 2 cups of caffeinated beverages. They must be consumed black and not contain dairy or any sweetener (artificial or natural)

- **You are encouraged to drink as much water throughout the day as you can manage, with an aim to meet 64 oz./2 litre goal.**

- You may drink the following herbal teas , either hot or cold, in unlimited quantities:
  - Lemon Balm
  - Green tea (decaf)
  - Peppermint
  - Dandelion

  ⇒ Use glucose regulating spices such as cinnamon and turmeric to avoid sugar cravings.
  ⇒ If you simply cannot do plain water, you can infuse water with fruit or vegetables. Just don't eat them.

⇒ DO NOT consume any sugar free sweet tasting drink, popsicles or jello.
⇒ Continue with your supplement routine.
⇒ Ensure you continue to take any prescribed medications.

End your day: By taking your probiotic before bed to allow it to colonize the GI tract.

Express Gratitude and Thanks

The trick to changing a lifetime of poor eating and the associated guilt that goes along with it is being thankful for the successes on your journey so fat and expressing gratitude and appreciation for your life and the things that come with it.

 Along this journey it is easy to feel lost, alone, resentful and guilty of our human failings. With that, feelings of overwhelm can creep in.

So, why not start a Gratitude Journal or Jar of Thanks.

Every day make a point to write down in your journal, or on a small piece of paper and put in your jar, one thing that you are grateful for that day.

Write down one thing you are proud of or one thing you have achieved.

Write down one thing and pop it in your jar, as many time a day as you feel appreciative or recognisant of the positive.

And when life starts giving you lemons, you can look in your journal or in your jar and see the delightful recipe to make lemonade with all the positive that is in your life.

It is a great way of changing your mindset and to shift your focus.

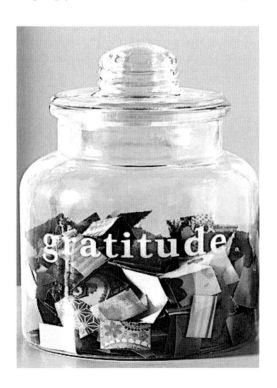

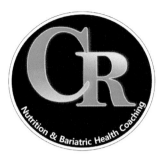

Fresh Start

Vegan / Vegetarian

Reset

DAY	INSTRUCTION "HOW TO EAT"	SELF-ASSESSMENT "What Homework task?"
1-2	Follow **Vegan Reset.** **Days 1-2 Instructions**	Follow **Original Reset Homework :** Days 1-2
3-7	Follow **Vegan Reset.** **Days 3-7 Instructions**	Follow **Original Reset Homework :** Days 3-7
8-14	Follow **Vegan Reset.** **Days 8-14 Instructions**	Follow **Original Reset Homework :** 8-14

Good luck on your journey, we will see you at the finish line.

Days 1 – 2

To start your day :

· 1 –2 tsp Apple Cider Vinegar (with the mother) in 1/4 cup of water (or)
· 1/2 cup raw organic Kombucha or Water Kefir.

Breakfast smoothie–

- 1 cup almond or coconut milk
- 1/2 cup berries such as blueberries or raspberries
- 1 handful baby spinach leaves (approx. 1/2 cup)
- 1 scoop of hemp or pea protein powder (equiv. 1 serve)
- 1/4 tsp. cinnamon
- Sweetener (to taste) (stevia or monk fruit)

Make up a big pot of Vegetable broth :

- Cabbage, Kale, Onion, Garlic, Carrot, celery, red peppers, turnip, Parsnip and sweet potato. Add spices like pink Himalayan salt, pepper, turmeric, chili etc.
- Soak 1-2 cups of dried Shitake mushrooms in 4 cups boiling water for 60 mins. Pour mushroom stock into vegetable broth and keep mushrooms for dinner recipe days 3 onwards.
- Simmer soup for a few hours, when all vegetables tender, take out any unwanted pieces and blend smooth.

- pescatarians can add fish stock to their broth.

- You can have up to 8 cups, if you do not drink all 8 cups, replace with another fluid like herbal tea or water.
- Ensure you are taking your vitamins
- Drink a min of 64 oz./2 litres of combined fluids (includes broth and tea etc).
- Take Probiotic of evening.

Days 3−7

<u>**To start your day :**</u>

· 1 −2 tsp Apple Cider Vinegar (with the mother) in 1/4 cup of water (or)
· 1/2 cup raw organic Kombucha or Water Kefir.

<u>**BREAKFAST:**</u>

- Protein smoothie (from day 1-2)
- **(OR)**
- 3 oz silken tofu (scrambled) with ;
    - 1/2 cup spinach (uncooked measure) sautéed
    - 1/4 cup sautéed mushrooms. (salt , pepper and garlic etc)

<u>**Throughout the day:**</u> Vegetable soup , up to 4 cups.

<u>**DINNER:**</u>

- RECIPE: Shitake Mushroom & Bean Burger with Salad/ or Veg.
- Or Store bought organic vegan patty.

   (OR)

- Firm Tofu & Vegetable Stir Fry

<u>**Pescatarians can alternate with:**</u>

4 oz. piece of protein. Fish (white fish, salmon or shrimp)
- With 3 oz. of green veg, any low carb green veg.

- Ensure you are taking your vitamins
- Drink a min of 64 oz./2 litres of combined fluids (includes broth and tea etc).
- Take Probiotic of evening.

Days 8 — 14

<u>**To start your day :**</u>
- 1 –2 tsp Apple Cider Vinegar (with the mother) in 1/4 cup of water (or)
- 1/2 cup raw organic Kombucha or Water Kefir.

<u>**BREAKFAST :**</u>
- Protein Smoothie (OR)
- Tofu Scramble (OR)
- 1/4 cup Vegan Yoghurt with 1/4 cup berries and 2 tbsp nuts

<u>**Morning Snack:**</u> Choose from snack list

<u>**LUNCH :**</u>

Option 1: Chickpea, apple and walnut salad.
- 2 tbsp drained chickpeas - 2 tbsp crushed walnuts - 1/2 diced apple - 1 cup baby spinach - 1 tbsp sunflower seeds - 1 large stalk celery chopped - Dressed with 2 tsp olive oil, 2 tsp apple cider vinegar, 2 tsp lemon juice, salt and pepper to taste.

Option 2: Stuffed Baked Capsicum Peppers (can also be a dinner option)
- Make a mix of 2 tbsp chick peas or lentils, 1/4 cup broad beans, chopped onion, grated carrot, tomato, chili, olive oil, salt, garlic and herbs. Stuff peppers and bake. * you can add 1 serve of hemp or pea protein to the mix.
- Pescatarians can choose to add fish, crab or shrimp to salad.

<u>**Afternoon Snack:**</u> Choose from snack list.

<u>**DINNER:**</u>
- Option 1: Shitake & Bean Burgers with salad or Veg
- Option 2: Firm Tofu or Tempeh stir fry.
- Option 3: Hearty Curry Veg Soup. (simply add more cubed veg to your broth adding 1/4 cup red lentils, your preferred curry spices and a dash of coconut cream)
- Pescatarian Option: White fish Curry or Fish and Vegetables

- Continue Supplement and Probiotic routine as normal.

SNACK LIST

- 1 cup of vegetable soup

- A cup cauliflower florets with 2 tbsp Hummus

- 1/4 cup vegan yoghurt with Strawberries

- 1/2 an avocado

- 20 almonds + 1/2 cup Strawberries

- 1/2 cup Grapes

- 1 oz Vegan Cheese with sundried tomatoes on cucumber slices.

- 1 large wedge of cantaloupe

- 1 medium wedge of watermelon

- 1/2 apple with nut butter

- 2 stalks of celery with nut butter

- Carrot sticks (1 small carrot) and 1 tbsp hummus

- Cup of Air-fried Kale chips

- 1/2 cup Avocado chocolate Chia pudding

- 1 cup of broccoli florets sautéed with sesame oil

Shitake Mushroom, Broad Bean & Hemp Burgers

Ready in 20

Each Patty has:

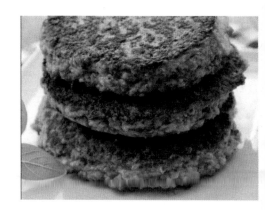

90 kcal	6.8 g Protein	2.5 g Fat	10 g Carbs

Ingredients

- 1 –2 cups soaked and drained Shitake mushrooms

- 1/2 cup frozen Broad Beans (Fava beans)

- 1/2 cup drained tinned chickpeas

- 1/2 cup hemp protein

- 1/4 cup frozen peas

- 1/4 cup frozen Corn

- 2 tbsp Nutritional yeast flakes

- 2 tsp coconut aminos

- 1 tbsp peanut butter

- Salt, Pepper, garlic

Instructions

Add all ingredients to a food processor and pulse until a thick and slightly chunky paste is achieved. If too wet, you can add a scoop or two of hemp protein. Add oil to a pan, and heat up.

Quickly form patties and Fry off on both sides. Place fried patties on a lined baking tray and bake in oven at approx. 300°F/ 160°C for a further 10-15 minutes until firm.

Reframe your thinking

Create a vision board.

If the imminent change, the immediate or distant future, the prospect of diet upheaval and trying to alter the course of your health and weight loss seems daunting and scary, try changing the thoughts about what lies ahead.

Sometimes the mere act of setting concrete goals can take the edge off anxiety about the dark and sinister future unknowns.

A good way to dispel the fear of the unknown is to spend a few hours collecting imagery from magazines and computer searches and even from Pinterest.

Write words of meaning on to stick-it notes and put it all together in the form of a vision board.

A vision board puts your thoughts fears and gaols all in one tangible, visible space and helps you gain clarity and focus.

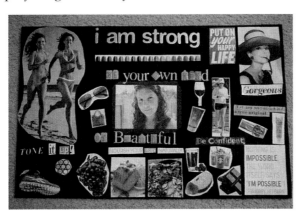

You could even try dividing the card into two, and on the left write or visually represent your goals (or both) with the statement at the top

"WHEN I ACHIEVE".

And on the right, "I WILL FEEL...", and again write or visually represent the culmination of your goals.

Having a clear direction of the path ahead, helps you keep moving when you stumble.

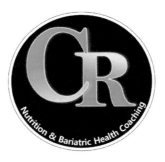

Fresh Start

Hypo-Glycaemic Control

&

Diabetes Support

Reset

DAY	INSTRUCTION "HOW TO EAT"	SELF-ASSESSMENT "What Homework task?"
1-2	Follow **Hypo Reset.** **Days 1-2 Instructions**	Follow **Original Reset Homework :** Days 1-2
3-7	Follow **Hypo Reset.** **Days 3-7 Instructions**	Follow **Original Reset Homework :** Days 3-7
8-14	Follow **Hypo Reset.** **Days 8-14 Instructions**	Follow **Original Reset Homework :** 8-14

Good luck on your journey, we will see you at the finish line.

Days 1 – 2

To start your day :

1 –2 tsp Apple Cider Vinegar (with the mother) in 1/4 cup of water (or)

1/2 cup raw organic Kombucha or Water Kefir.

Breakfast smoothie–
- 1 cup almond milk
- 1/2 cup berries
- 1 handful baby spinach leaves
- 1 scoop of low carb vanilla protein powder
- 1/4 tsp. cinnamon

(OR)
- 2 scrambled eggs with 1 tbsp cream cheese and 1/2 cup spinach (uncooked measure) sautéed.

(OR)
- 1 piece of bacon, 1 egg and sautéed mushrooms.

- Make up a big pot of Bone broth as per the recipe in the book:
- You can have up to 6 cups, if you do not drink all 6 cups, replace with another fluid like herbal tea or water.

For lunch on both days:

A green salad consisting of lettuce, spinach, 1 tbsp of sunflower seeds/ or pepitas, 1 tbsp crushed walnuts, 1/2 a chopped apple, 1 tsp raisins and 1 stalk of celery chopped. You can add some light oil if you wish .

For Dinner on Both days:

A small fillet of white fish or Chicken, grilled. Served with green beans and /or Broccoli. (approx. 3 oz/85g size fillet) approx. 6 –8 green beans and/ OR 3 broccoli flowerets

- Ensure you are taking your vitamins,
- Drink a min of 64 oz./2 litres of combined fluids (includes broth and tea etc).
- Take Probiotic of evening.

Days 3—7

<u>**To start your day :**</u>

1 –2 tsp Apple Cider Vinegar (with the mother) in 1/4 cup of water (or)

1/2 cup raw organic Kombucha or Water Kefir.

<u>**BREAKFAST:**</u>

- Protein smoothie (from day 1-2)

<u>**(OR)**</u>

- 1/2 Cup Greek yoghurt (no sugar) with 1 tbsp crush almonds/walnuts, some mixed berries.

<u>**(OR)**</u>

- Scrambled eggs with Cream cheese and spinach.

<u>**MORNING SNACK:**</u>

Broth/ Vegetable soup (can have some small veg pieces i.e. 1 – 2 tbsp of chopped carrot, celery, green bean)

<u>**LUNCH:**</u>

2-3oz. Protein with 2 oz. salad/veg

Example : • tuna lettuce cups • Steak and salad • Bun less burger w/salad • Chicken veg stir-fry

<u>**AFTERNOON SNACK :**</u>

Broth/ Vegetable soup (can have some small veg pieces i.e. 1 –2 tbsp of chopped carrot, celery, green bean) - a good soup recipe is Atkins Turbo Soup (google)

<u>**DINNER:**</u>

3 –4 oz. piece of protein. Fish (white fish, salmon or shrimp) (or) chicken. With 3 oz. of green veg, any low carb green veg.

Days 8 — 14

<u>To start your day :</u>

1 –2 tsp Apple Cider Vinegar (with the mother) in 1/4 cup of water (or)

1/2 cup raw organic Kombucha or Water Kefir.

<u>STRUCTURE:</u> **Breakfast> Morning Snack> Lunch> Afternoon Snack> Dinner**

<u>BREAKFAST:</u> Not to exceed 1 cup in total.

Must contain • Protein and some small amount of carbs

Examples:

- 1/4 cup Yoghurt with berries and nuts
- Protein shake with berries and almond milk
- 2 fried eggs, with spinach and mushroom
- 2oz protein and veg (chicken and veg from leftovers)

<u>SNACK:</u>   One item from the list.

<u>LUNCH:</u>

Must contain

- 2-3 oz. of Protein
- 1 cup of salad (or) 3/4 cup of cooked vegetables
- 1-2 tsp of fats

<u>SNACK:</u>   One item from the list

<u>DINNER</u>

Must contain

- 3-4 oz. of Protein (and no more)
- 1 cup of salad (or) 3/4 cup of cooked vegetables
- 1-2 tsp of fats
- You can include a small amount of gravy or sauce to your dinner meals too.

SNACK LIST

- 1 cup Bone Broth + 1 oz. Shredded Chicken

- A cup cauliflower florets with 2 tbsp Hummus

- 10 almonds + 6 Strawberries

- 1 medium wedge of Watermelon or Cantaloupe

- 2 stalks of celery with nut butter

- Cup of Air-fried Kale chips.

- 1 cup of broccoli florets sautéed with sesame oil

- Half a boiled egg in a lettuce leaf with ¼ avocado

  + 1 tsp of real egg mayo

- 6 slices of cucumber, cream cheese/cottage cheese or feta
  (1 tsp on each) and 2 slices of ham divided into 6.

- 10 green beans with a tbsp. of Persian feta or chopped dill
  pickle mixed with cream cheese

- 1 oz. of chicken or turkey breast with 4-6 cheddar cheese cubes.

- ¼ cup blueberries and 10 almonds or pistachios

- 2 roll ups – e.g. salami/pepperoni wrapped around any
  deli cheese like mozzarella, provolone, cheddar

- 2 bacon wrapped asparagus spears

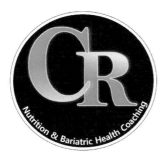

Fresh Start

Exercise & Workout Support

Reset

DAY	INSTRUCTION "HOW TO EAT"	SELF-ASSESSMENT "What Homework task?"
1-2	Follow **Exercise Support Reset.** **Days 1-2 Instructions**	Follow **Original Reset** **Homework :** Days 1-2
3-7	Follow **Exercise Support Reset.** **Days 3-7 Instructions**	Follow **Original Reset** **Homework :** Days 3-7
8-14	Follow **Exercise Support Reset.** **Days 8-14 Instructions**	Follow **Original Reset** **Homework :** 8-14

Good luck on your journey, we will see you at the finish line.

Days 1 – 2

<u>**To start your day**</u> :

1 –2 tsp Apple Cider Vinegar (with the mother) in 1/4 cup of water (or)

1/2 cup raw organic Kombucha or Water Kefir.

<u>**BREAKFAST:**</u>

<u>Simple Protein Shake</u>

- 1 cup almond milk
- 1 scoop of low carb vanilla protein powder (whey or hemp)

<u>**SNACKS:**</u>

- Make up a big pot of Bone broth as per the recipe in the book:
- You can have up to 6 cups, if you do not drink all 6 cups, replace with another fluid like herbal tea or water.

<u>**FOR LUNCH ON BOTH DAYS:**</u>

- 1 cup of Steamed Broccoli
- 1 simple protein shake .

<u>**FOR DINNER ON BOTH DAYS:**</u>

- A small fillet of white fish or Chicken, grilled.
- Served with 1/2-1cup green beans and /or Broccoli.

- Ensure you are taking your bariatric vitamins,
- Drink a min of 64 oz./2 litres of combined fluids (includes broth and tea etc).
- Take Probiotic of evening.

Days 3–7

<u>To start your day :</u>

     1 –2 tsp Apple Cider Vinegar (with the mother) in 1/4 cup of water (or)

     1/2 cup raw organic Kombucha or Water Kefir.

BREAKFAST:

Simple Protein Shake

- 1 cup almond milk
- 1 scoop of low carb vanilla protein powder (whey or hemp)

MORNING SNACK:

- 1 Cup bone broth with/ 1.oz shredded chicken and 1 small handful of spinach greens.

LUNCH:

- 3 oz. Tuna or chicken
- 1-2 cups salad leaves
- 2 tsp olive oil

AFTERNOON SNACK :

- 1 Cup bone broth with/ 1.oz shredded chicken and 1 small handful of spinach greens.

DINNER:

- A small fillet of white fish or Chicken, grilled.
- Served with 1/2-1cup green beans and /or Broccoli.

- Ensure you are taking your bariatric vitamins,
- Drink a min of 64 oz./2 litres of combined fluids (includes broth and tea etc).
- Take Probiotic of evening.

Days 8 — 14

<u>**To start your day :**</u>

> 1 –2 tsp Apple Cider Vinegar (with the mother) in 1/4 cup of water (or)

> 1/2 cup raw organic Kombucha or Water Kefir.

<u>Breakfast> Morning Snack> Lunch> Afternoon Snack> Dinner</u>

<u>**BREAKFAST:**</u>   Not to exceed 1 cup in total.

- 1/4 cup Greek Yoghurt with berries and nuts (OR)
- 2 fried eggs, with spinach and mushroom (OR)
- 2oz protein and veg (chicken and veg from leftovers)

<u>**MORNING SNACK:**</u>

- 1 simple protein shake .

<u>**LUNCH:**</u>

- 3 oz. Chicken/Fish, grilled.
- 1 cup of Steamed Broccoli (OR) 1-2 cups Salad Leaves
- 1 tbsp crushed Almonds
- 2 tsp Olive oil.

<u>**AFTERNOON SNACK :**</u>   One item from the SNACK list

<u>**DINNER:**</u>

- 4 oz. white fish or Chicken, grilled.
- 1 cup of Steamed Broccoli/Green beans (OR) 1-2 cups Salad Leaves
- 1-2 tsp olive oil or grass fed butter
- Spices if you wish
- You can include a small amount of gravy or sauce. Ensure you are taking your bariatric vitamins,
- Drink a min of 64 oz./2 litres of combined fluids (includes broth/ tea etc).
- Take Probiotic of evening.

"I am transforming into someone who is happy and positive."

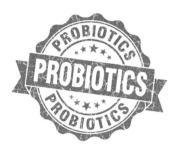

Studies have been conducted into the correlations between the gut biome and obesity . The changes in the biome due to highly stressed, over medicated and high sugar lifestyles, allow bad (non indigenous) bacteria to flourish and leads us down the path to ill health.

It would therefore appear that healthy gut microbiota are equally important in weight loss after surgery.

Probiotics are essentially the helpful micro-organisms that live and thrive in our intestines. They have a variety of influences on our internal systems ranging from digestive processes to immune functions, production of vitamins and fatty acids and keep the bad bacteria within healthy limits.

There have been some very promising studies that have revealed that the use of probiotic supplements after Gastric Bypass and associated bariatric surgeries, promoted better outcomes to patients' weight loss and nutritional profiles (as in levels of micro-nutrients in the body).

The Gut Brain Connection

Our gut does more than help us digest food; the bacteria that call our intestines home have been implicated in everything from our mental health and sleep, to weight gain and cravings for certain foods.

A recent study found that the addition of a "good" strain of the bacteria lactobacillus (which is also found in yoghurt) to the gut of normal mice reduced their anxiety levels. The effect was blocked after cutting the Vagus nerve (which is the main nerve to the stomach and the main connection between brain and gut). This suggests the gut-brain axis is being used by bacteria to affect the brain.

- This connection was further clarified in a study where bacterial metabolites (by-products) from fibre digestion were found to increase the levels of the gut hormone and neurotransmitter, serotonin. Serotonin can activate the vagus nerve. This suggests one way your gut bacteria might be linked with your brain. Therefore low serotonin (as seen in anxiety and depression) can cause cravings to 'feed your bacteria' - (and they feed off sugars).

- Interestingly, in two human studies that looked at people with major depression; it was found that the bacteria in their faeces differed from healthy non-depressed volunteers. Therefore it was concluded that changes to gut bacteria from antibiotics are associated with anxious and depressive behaviours.

A good quality probiotic may help to:

- Improve Serotonin production and absorption.

- Promote more effective carbohydrate metabolism.

- Support fatigue, by enhancing restorative sleep.

- Enhance overall nutrient levels.

- Support nutrient absorption.

- Aid in the digestion of dairy and ease digestive discomfort.

- Re-establish gut flora after antibiotic use.

- Stimulate immune system to fight bacterial infections.

- Lower allergy response and inflammation.

- Decrease symptoms of Leaky Gut Syndrome, IBS, and constipation.

- Improve allergy and Hay Fever.

- Break down complex carbohydrates, fat and protein into small components, thus increasing absorption of vital nutrients.

- Prevent the growth of bad bacteria and yeasts.

Supporting your gut is Supporting your goal.

BARIATRIC SUPPLEMENT GUIDE

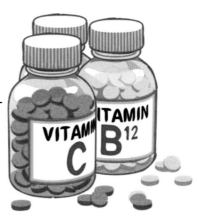

You should have all been made aware by your surgeon/ bariatric GP, dietician etc., that weight loss surgery can and will cause issues relating to malabsorption which can lead to widespread vitamin and mineral deficiency.

This can present itself as brittle hair and nails, loss of dental integrity and lost teeth, fatigue, loss of mental acuity, just to name a few.

The enzymes needed for the proper breakdown of the foods that we eat are produced in the first portion of the digestive tract, being our mouths and stomach. Some of the nutrients we ingest are absorbed by the villi (finger like projections) that line our stomachs, and much of absorption takes place in the first third of the small intestine (duodenum and jejunum).

Weight loss surgeries such as Gastric Sleeve, reduce the size of the stomach thereby reducing the absorptive surface of the stomach (less villi), RNY not only reduces the size of the stomach drastically but it bypasses the duodenum, so food we ingest does not go through its main absorption channel.

We lose weight due to this limited capacity, and limited absorption, as we absorb less calories, yet in turn we absorb less nutrient and minerals too.

Liquid emptying occurs prior to solid emptying, that's why we must wait before we drink, to give our food a chance to digest, and reduce chances of dumping – which does not allow anything to be absorbed.

Therefore, it is very important to implement and stick to a well-balanced supplement protocol early on.

Bariatric Supplement Guide

	It is important to include the supplements highlighted in Green as a minimum.	
Supplement	ACTIONS	How much & When?
Complex Multi-V	Multivitamins should consist of all the basics, vitamins A, C and E, vitamin D and magnesium, potassium, and other essential minerals. Try and find a multi that contains B1 (Thiamine). Thiamine is not stored in the body and must be consumed daily. It's essential for the conversion of carbohydrates into energy, and it's necessary for brain and nerve cell function.	Dependant on the quality of your multi, a single daily morning dose should be sufficient.
Calcium Citrate	Calcium plays an important role in the body. It is essential in preventing bone loss, osteoporosis, parathyroid dysfunction and is important in muscle contraction. If you do not get enough dietary calcium, your body will begin to leach calcium from your bones and teeth to carry out its functions. Take in conjunction with vitamin D as D is essential in calcium absorption. * Stay away from 'CHEWS', anything that is gummy or chewy is made with glucose.	1,200-1,500 mg daily. *TIP* Buy a Vitamin D and Cal Citrate combo.
Vitamin D	Is essential for bone mineralisation and both Calcium and magnesium absorption. It plays a huge role in mental health and immune function. Important for fertility and overall general health.	At least 1000- 2000 IU Vitamin D per day. *TIP* Take with your fish oil or dietary fats as Vitamin D is Fat soluble.
Probiotic	Probiotics are live bacteria and yeasts that are good for your health, especially your digestive system. They help to break down and convert the foods that we eat into usable proteins and energy. Probiotics aid motility, can aid in the treatment of IBD/IBS, antibiotic related yeast infections, yeast overgrowth (thrush), reduce allergy symptoms, aid in oral health and improve skin conditions. You are looking for live strain probiotic that has a minimum 10 million CFUs per dose.	Double dose every night for 1 month, then 1 dose per night ongoing. *TIP* Taken at night before bed as the LAST thing you ingest to allow them time to colonise the GI tract. *** DID YOU KNOW THAT 95% OF OUR SEROTONIN IS IN THE GASTROINTESTINAL TRACT?**
B12	Vitamin B12 is a powerhouse. It helps make DNA, nerve and blood cells, and is crucial for a healthy brain and immune system. Look for Sublingual (under the tongue) Activated B12 or **METHYLCOBALAMIN ONLY** Cyanocobalamin is NOT bio-available and therefore not absorbed.	1,000 mcg daily

Iron & Folate	Especially important for women of childbearing age and pre-menopausal women. Iron deficiency is especially prevalent in RNY patients due to the limited gastric capacity. Vitamin C is recommended in conjunction with Iron to increase absorption. Heme iron (meat sourced iron) is most readily absorbed. Iron and folate are important for energy, mental clarity, oxygen saturation and healing, as well as MANY other important functions. Iron deficiency anaemia is very common in those who have undergone WLS.	15-20 mg per day of iron 400-600 mcg of folate per day. *TIP* A pregnancy and breastfeeding iron/folate formula will meet these needs
Vitamin C	Vitamin C is an important vitamin and antioxidant that the body uses to keep you strong and healthy. Vitamin C is used in the maintenance of bones, muscle, and blood vessels. Vitamin C also assists in the formation of collagen and helps the body absorb iron.	100mg a day minimum
DHA and EPA Omega 3's & 6's (Fish Oil)	The omega-3 fatty acid docosahexaenoic acid (DHA) is crucial for the healthy structure and function of the brain. An optimal intake of DHA is especially essential for pregnant and nursing mothers to ensure adequate brain development in their children. Helps relieve pain and inflammation, stimulates skin and hair growth. Fatty acids both supplemental and dietary are CRUCIAL for all nervous system functions.	2 x 1000 mg capsules daily. *TIP* take with your Vitamin D to aid in absorption. *TIP* Cod-liver Oil is a great source of Omega 3s & 6's, as well as Vitamin A and Vitamin D.
Magnesium	Magnesium is a nutrient that the body needs to stay healthy. Magnesium is important for many processes in the body, including regulating muscle and nerve function, blood sugar levels, and blood pressure and making protein, bone, and DNA. Magnesium aids sleep, and can help lessen the pain associated with muscle cramping, Fibromyalgia and Rheumatic disorders. Low magnesium also plays a role in KETO FLU, so make sure you get enough of this vital nutrient to help avoid it! Magnesium malate is the most natural and easily absorbed form of Magnesium so find a Mg Malate supplement.	Before bed 350 mg *TIP* magnesium competes with iron and zinc for absorption, so take it on its own before bed and help your sleep too. *adding your magnesium powder to hot beverages ionises the compounds making them more bio-available and therefore better absorbed.

Biotin	Biotin, or Vitamin B7, is a water-soluble vitamin that's a part of the vitamin B complex — a group of key nutrients needed for healthy metabolic, nerve, digestive and cardiovascular functions. Hair loss and brittle nails may have multiple causes and taking biotin supplements **may** help this process. **However studies have shown that a balanced diet has far greater effect , and that we get our RDI of Biotin from our daily diet, so its up to you but generally unnecessary.**	2.5 mg (or 2,500 mcg) *Studies have suggested that Supplemental Biotin can interfere with certain pathology results. So the cessation of biotin is recommended more than 72 hours prior to scheduled bloods.
Prebiotic Fibre	Pre-biotic fibres are non-digestible plant fibres that feed your bacteria, they promote the growth of beneficial microorganisms in the intestines and the more food, or prebiotics, that probiotics have to eat, the more efficiently these live bacteria work and the healthier your gut will be. There are Pre-biotic fibres such as psyllium husk/ psyllium husk powder, raw garlic, raw dandelion green, to name a few. You can also buy a pre-biotic supplement to take daily.	5 g of prebiotic fibre per day.
L-Glutamine	Is an amino acid that is not only essential in protein synthesis, but it also aid in muscle repair, especially the smooth muscular walls of your GI tract. The better our GI health, the better our absorption. You can take Glutamine in powder or tablet form or alternatively, cabbage water/cabbage broth is an excellent dietary source – you can make bone broth with cabbage and get a tonne of nutrients.	This usually comes in powdered form with serving size of 5 g (1 tsp.).
Chromium	Chromium is used to regulate blood sugar and therefore can be a useful supplement to aid in the reduction of sugar cravings.	250mcg per day
Zinc	Is important for healing and immune function. Especially important for males as it is vital for reproductive health and sperm production.	10 mg

Supplements in Blue are recommended to meet optimal levels as per Nationally suggested RDIs, and are not intended to replace the advice of your GP and do not endorse the cessation of any prescribed medications.

Please seek advice from your doctor if something is not right for you.

Content provided in this book is of a general nature only and does not replace the information and advice provided by your own health care professionals. Always consult your own health providers for specific personal health and medical advice.

128

Recipes

For Low-Carb Living when you transition
to the Balanced Macros Program

Recipes for Low-Carb Living

on the

Balanced Macros Program

Cinnamon Roll
Pork Cracklings

Ready in 2 min

A 0.5 oz. /20g Serve has:

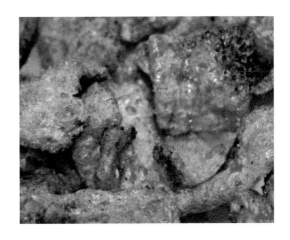

85.7	7.02 g	6.28 g	1 g
kcal	Protein	Fat	Carbs

Ingredients

1 LARGE bag of Pork rinds (Pork crackle/Chicharrones)

4 T. butter, melted

1 T. cinnamon

1-2 tsp. powdered sweetener

Instructions

Place pork rinds in an extra large ziploc bag.

Pour melted butter over pork rinds.

Close bag and shake until pork rinds are coated in butter.

Mix together cinnamon and sweetener, sprinkle over pork rinds, shake bag again until pork rinds are coated in cinnamon mixture.

Store in air-tight container.

Savoury Cheese & Tofu Muffins

Each muffin contains:

127 kcal	10 g Protein	9 g Fat	2 g Carbs

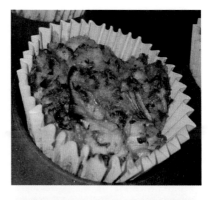

Ingredients

6 Medium eggs

2 Tbsp. Oil – Olive or any nut oil.

10 g, Tuscan Seasoning

30 g, Parmesan grated

1 medium Leek sliced

15 g, Minced Garlic

2 x Chicken Stock Cubes

4 large strips of Bacon

150 g, Cheese, cheddar grated

500 g, Organic Tofu, Firm and crumbled

1 container (247.50 gram), Chopped Spinach (frozen)

Salt and Pepper

3 Tbsp. Psyllium husk

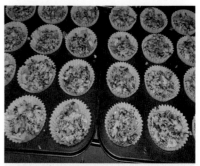

Instructions

Pre-heat your oven to 180'C/360'F

Its as simple as adding everything to a bowl, crumbling the tofu, chopping the bacon, adding the eggs and mixing together.

Use cupcake trays and patty cases, divide he mix into 24 (approx. 1 heaped tbsp. of wet mix per patty case) Bake for approx. 20 minutes until golden and firm.

Let cool and enjoy.

Put cooled muffins in a Ziploc bag and freeze for convenience

Cauliflower Crispy Dippers

Ready in 45 min.

Each Dipper has:

40	3.83 g	2.34 g	1.5 g
kcal	Protein	Fat	Carbs

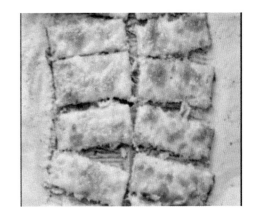

Ingredients

1 head cauliflower washed, dried or 4 cups chopped

1/4 cup grated Parmesan cheese

1 egg

1 teaspoon Italian seasonings

1 teaspoon garlic powder

1/2 teaspoon salt

1 1/2 cup mozzarella cheese shredded

Instructions

Preheat oven to 425 degrees.

Line 2 baking trays with baking paper.

Cut cauliflower into bite size pieces steam for 20 minutes until just tender.

Place cauliflower in food processor and pulse until the size of rice.

Pour riced cauliflower into a large bowl and add Parmesan cheese, egg, seasonings and 1/2 cup mozzarella cheese. Mix well then spread mixture tray in a rectangle.

Bake for 10-15 minutes until browned on top. Invert over Turn out onto other baking tray. Sprinkle mozzarella over the top and bake another 5-10 minutes until browned.

Let rest 10 minutes. Slice into 24 pieces.

Mini Chipotle, Cheese, Bacon and Broccoli Frittatas

Ready in 30 minutes

Each frittata has:

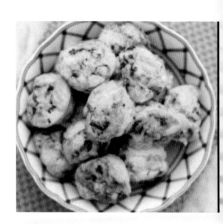

66 kcal	5 g Protein	4 g Fat	1 g Carbs

Ingredients

1 1/2 cups chopped broccoli

12 eggs

2/3 cup water

1/2 tsp chipotle pepper powder

1/2 tsp salt

1 1/2 green onions (white & green parts), thinly sliced

1/3 cup grated Cheddar cheese

Instructions

Preheat oven to 375 degrees F. Prepare a 12-cup muffin tin by coating each cup with cooking spray. Set a medium saucepan of water over high heat and bring to a boil. Add broccoli and cook until just tender, about 1½ minutes. Drain and immediately rinse with cold water. In a large bowl, whisk together eggs, water, chipotle pepper powder, and kosher salt.

Divide the broccoli, green onions and cheddar cheese between the muffin tin cups.

Transfer the egg mixture to a bowl or measuring cup with a spout and pour the egg over the broccoli mixture, filling each cup to no more than ¾ full. Bake until the egg is set and the tops of the frittatas are starting to brown, 20 to 25 minutes. Run a knife or thin metal spatula around the edge of each frittata and gently lift them out. Serve immediately.

Sweet Poppers

Ready in 25 min.

Each popper has:

65	3 g	5 g	2.3g
kcal	Protein	Fat	Carbs

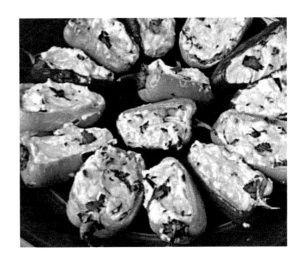

Ingredients

1 lb / 500g mini sweet peppers halved

8 ounces smoked Gouda cheese grated

8 ounces cream cheese room temperature

1/2 cup crumbled feta cheese

1/4 cup grated onion

2 cloves garlic minced

2 tablespoons chopped cilantro

Instructions

Preheat oven to 425 degrees.

In a bowl mix all ingredients together.

Fill each pepper half with mixture.

Bake 15-20 minutes until cheese is melted and slightly browned. And peppers have softened.

Creamy Cauliflower NO -TATOE Mash

Ready in 30 min.

A 2 oz. / 60g serving is

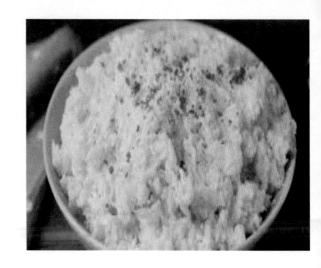

43.12	1,19 g	3 44 g	2 64 g
kcal	Protein	Fat	Carbs

Ingredients

1 Large head of Cauliflower, 1.22 head (703 g)

3 tbsp. Cream Cheese, 1.5 ounces (42 g)

2 tbsp. Salted Butter, 0.13 cup (28 g)

Heavy Cream, 0.12 cup (28 g)

Salt and White pepper - to taste,1 teaspoon (5 g)

Instructions

Chop cauliflower into small pieces, and boil until soft.

When soft drain well and add back to saucepan.

Mash with butter, cream cheese, cream, salt and pepper.

Use stick blender to make smooth.

Stir over heat to remove excess moisture.

Use as a side-dish accompaniment to any meal .

Garlic Mustard Greens

Ready in 10 minutes

A 2 oz./ 60g serving has

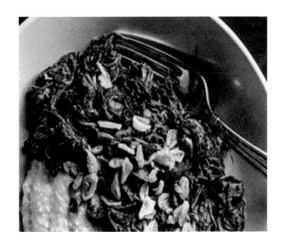

21	1.85 g	0.26 g	3.94 g Carbs

Ingredients

2 tablespoons extra-virgin olive oil

6 large garlic cloves, thinly sliced

2 bunches (1 1/2 lbs. total) mustard greens, leaves torn into bite-size pieces and stems discarded

1 teaspoon raw cane sugar or agave nectar

1 teaspoon coarse sea salt, divided

2 tablespoons red wine vinegar

Instructions

Bring a large pot of water, seasoned with 1/2 tsp. salt, to a boil. Meanwhile, fill a sink or bowl with cold water.

Boil mustard greens until bright green, about 2 minutes. Drain well and press to remove as much liquid as possible. Set aside.

Heat garlic and oil together in frying pan over medium heat until garlic is   golden and fragrant, 5 to 7 minutes.

Use a slotted spoon to transfer the garlic chips to a plate.

Raise heat to high and quickly add sugar, remaining 1/2 tsp. salt, and the   vinegar. Cook until sugar dissolves, about 3 minutes. Add reserved mustard greens and stir to coat.

Cook until most of the liquid is gone, about 3 minutes. Serve greens over cauli mash with a sprinkle of garlic chips.

Roasted NO-TATOES (radishes)

Ready in 30 min.

A 2 oz. /60 g serve (approx. 3 pieces) has:

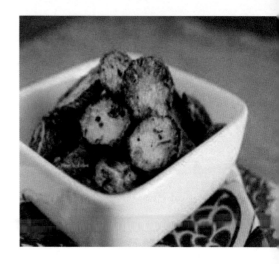

74 kcal	0.63 g Protein	7.04 g Fat	2.84 g Carbs

Ingredients

8 cups radishes, trimmed and halved

8 garlic cloves, minced

Tbsp. grass-fed butter or ghee, melted

1 tsp. sea salt

1 tsp. pepper

Optional fresh parsley, dill or chives

Instructions

Preheat oven to 400 degrees.

Line a roasting pan or baking tray with foil and set aside.

Clean and trim radishes, cut into halves.

Combine all ingredients in a bowl and toss so that the radishes are evenly   coated with the mixture.

Place radishes cut side down on tray.

Bake until slightly golden, approx. 15mins .

Garnish with fresh chopped herbs i.e. parsley, dill, chives, cilantro/coriander. Serve with sour cream or low carb gravy

Green Salad with Celery, Walnuts and Cranberries

Ready in 10 min.

A 2 oz. Serve has:

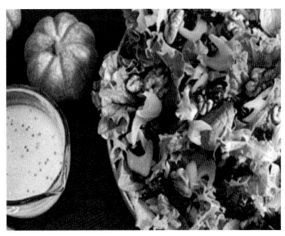

81 kcal	1.02 g Protein	6.15 g Fat	6 g Carbs

Ingredients

1/2 teaspoon salt

1/4 cup olive oil

1/2 cup dried cranberries

1 1/2 cups sliced celery (about 3 ribs)

1/2 cup walnuts, toasted

1 tablespoon honey

1/4 cup apple cider vinegar

1 tablespoon grainy mustard

10 cup mixed greens

1/4 teaspoon pepper

Instructions

Make dressing: Whisk cider, vinegar, honey and mustard. Slowly whisk in oil. Add salt and pepper.

Make salad: Place greens, celery, cranberries and walnuts in a bowl. Toss with just enough dressing to lightly coat.

Pass remaining dressing on the side.

Alfredo Creamed Spinach

Ready in 20 min.

A 2 oz. /60 g Serve has:

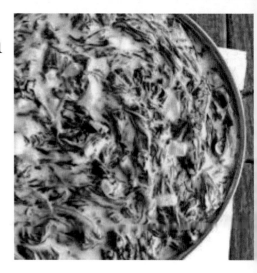

71 kcal	2.48 g Protein	5.99 g Fat	2.04 g Carbs

Ingredients

1/4 pound bacon strips, chopped,

frozen chopped spinach,20.7 oz

1 jar (15 ounces) alfredo sauce,15.2 oz

3/4 teaspoon pepper,0.1 oz

Instructions

Cook spinach according to package directions.

Meanwhile, in a large skillet, cook bacon over medium heat until crisp.

Remove to paper towels with a slotted spoon; drain, reserving 3 tablespoons drippings.

Drain spinach. In the same skillet, sauté spinach in reserved drippings for   1 minute. Stir in the alfredo sauce, pepper and bacon; heat through.

Roasted Brussels Sprouts with Ham and Garlic

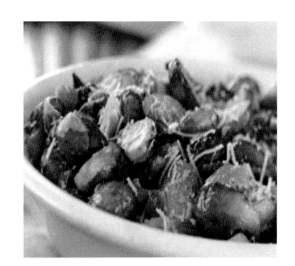

Ready in 45 min.

A 2 oz. / 60 g Serving has:

32 kcal	2.27 g Protein	0.68 g Fat	5.48 g Carbs

Ingredients

2 tablespoons grated fresh parmesan cheese

1/2 teaspoon salt

1 teaspoon olive oil

2 tablespoons fresh lemon juice

3 pounds Brussel sprouts, trimmed and halved

3 garlic cloves, thinly sliced

1 slice white bread

1/4 cup finely chopped country ham (about 1 ounce)

Instructions

Preheat oven to 425. Pulse bread in food, Sprinkle crumbs on a baking sheet; bake at 425 until golden. Reduce oven temperature to 375. Set aside 3 tablespoons toasted bread-crumbs.

Combine sprouts , garlic, lemon juice, olive oil, ham and salt on a baking dish coated with cooking spray, tossing to coat.

Bake for 30 minutes until sprouts are tender and lightly browned stirring twice. Sprinkle 3 tbsp. breadcrumbs and Parmesan cheese over sprouts.

German Green Beans

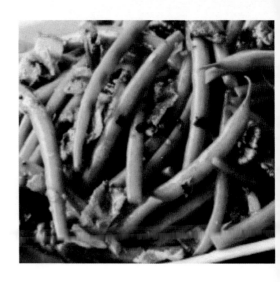

Ready in 30 min.

A 2 oz. / 60g serve has:

59.92 kcal	2.13 g Protein	4.38 g Fat	3.5 g Carbs

Ingredients

6 bacon strips

1-1/2 pounds fresh green beans, cut into 1-inch pieces

1 large onion, chopped

Salt and pepper to taste

Instructions

Place beans in a saucepan and cover with water; bring to a boil.

Reduce heat; cover and cook for 15-20 minutes or until tender.

Meanwhile, in a skillet, cook bacon until crisp. Remove bacon and set aside.

Sauté onion in drippings until tender; remove with a slotted spoon.

Drain beans; return to pan.

Add onion, 1 tablespoon drippings, salt and pepper; heat through.

Crumble the bacon; add to the beans and toss.

Serve immediately.

Bacon Cheese Chicken Roll Ups

Each Chicken roll up contains

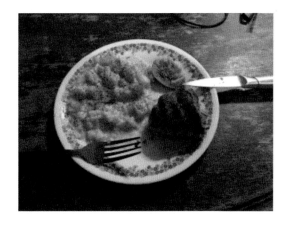

478 kcal	37.8 g Protein	34.5 g Fat	1.9 g Carbs

Ingredients

4 chicken breast small or 2 large chicken breasts

1 oz. mozzarella for each breast

Salt and pepper

Sprinkle of garlic powder for each or Italian seasonings

1 slice of pork bacon for each breast (turkey bacon will not work)

Optional low carb tomato sauce

Cotton twine or toothpicks

Instructions

Preheat oven to 350 degrees Fahrenheit

Pound out each chicken breast to me flat. Cut mozzarella into slices from ball. Set aside. Get seasonings out and set to side.

Take one breast and sprinkle with salt and pepper both sides, then one side with garlic powder or Italian seasoning. On the full seasoning side, layer cheese and roll up the chicken into a ball. Wrap bacon slice around the chicken roll up and tie with twine or stick it closed with a toothpick.

At this point you can freeze these to be cooked later for quick dinners. Wrap each one in plastic wrap and into a baggie and freeze.

Do not freeze the toothpick but twine can be frozen.

Bake until meat thermometer registers 160-180

Burger Stacks

Each stack contains

372 kcal	32 g Protein	25 g Fat	4 g Carbs

With Cheese

393 kcal	32 g Protein	27 g Fat	4 g Carbs

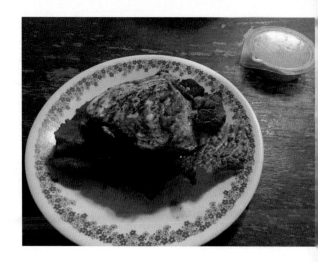

Ingredients

Hamburger patties

Guacamole

Salt and pepper

Lettuce

Cooked bacon strips pork or turkey

Crispy fried egg

Sour cream

Optional:

1/2 oz. Cheese

Instructions

Cook the Hamburger patties. Cook bacon. Cook the egg if using

On a plate put down a lettuce leaf or two, add the burger, layer on the guacamole, bacon and egg. Layer another leaf or two of lettuce and either wrap the burger to eat with hands or use a fork. The egg yolk creates a dressing for it almost.

Pot Stickers on a Stick

Each pot sticker contains

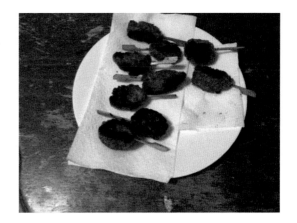

118	8.8 g	8.7 g	1.4 g
kcal	Protein	Fat	Carbs

Ingredients

1 pound ground pork

1 cup shredded green cabbage

3 oz. of chopped mushrooms

2 cloves of garlic, pressed or mashed

1 tbsp. grated ginger

1 tbsp. coconut aminos

Salt and pepper to taste

1 Tbsp. sesame oil

12 wooden kebob or canapé sticks , soaked

Instructions

Can be sautéed in a pan. If you cook in a pan do not add sesame oil to the meat! If you cook

this in the oven add sesame oil in the meat. Preheat oven to 350 and prepare a baking sheet with parchment or get out a pan for the stove.

Mix all the above in the bowl and form into 12 meat balls or form a sausage like shape and insert the wooden stick to cook.

Cook in oven for 20 min. Or pan fry in sesame oil until meat is done.

Make a dipping sauce of coconut aminos and sesame oil!

Quick and Dirty Cauliflower Bake

Approx. 6 Bari-Serve

Side Dish

56 kcal	3.8 g Protein	3.8 g Fat	1.2 g Carbs

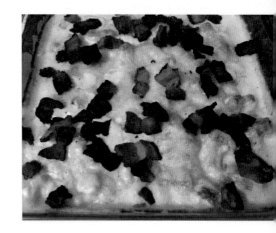

Ingredients

1 bag frozen cauliflower (400g)

1 cup shredded cheese

1/2 cup cream

1 to 1.5 cups of broth Beef/chicken/bone)

4 slices bacon

Instructions

Preheat oven to 350 degree Fahrenheit (180' C).

In an oven safe cast iron skillet or casserole dish (Pyrex), dump in frozen   cauliflower florets. Add salt and pepper.

In bowl mix cream, broth and cheese.

Pour over cauliflower and bake for 30-40 min. Cook bacon slices and cut or break apart.

When cauliflower is soft and cheese is bubbly take out of oven and sprinkle on bacon.

Recipe by: Jonica Kelly— Author of "Low-Carb, No-Fuss" (*Coming soon)

CBC Meatloaf (chicken, Bacon, cheese)

Each 3/4 inch slice has

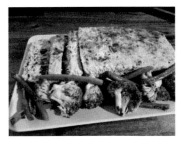

142 kcal	14 g Protein	8 g Fat	2 g Carbs

Ingredients

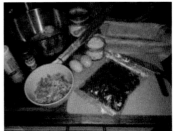

1/2 tsp. Salt , 1/2 tsp. ground white pepper

1 tsp. Tuscan Seasoning (Au) (mix of garlic, salt, rosemary, black pepper – or what ever flavors you like with chicken)

100 g, Grated Cheddar cheese

4 tsp, Crushed Garlic , 1 Leek, chopped finely

1 1/2 cups, Frozen Spinach

4 large rashers of Bacon, Diced

2 large Eggs

Half a Kilo/ 1 Lb. Chicken Mince Meat (defrosted)

Instructions

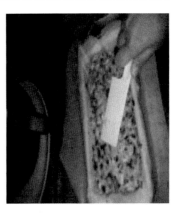

Add all ingredients to a mixing bowl and combine.

Once combined, you want to help the loaf hold together without using bread crumbs or any other high carb filler. You do this by manually breaking down the proteins. manually 'knead' the mixture in the bowl with a 'flip and push' motion, use force and allow the mix to be compacted with the motion. Do this for about a minute. You will notice that the mince take on a less grainy texture and more of a sticky texture.

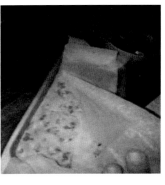

When combined and 'kneaded', pack the mixture into a standard 8" Loaf tin that has been lined with baking paper. Use enough baking paper that you have enough to fold over the top. Press the mix into the tin, and smooth out with a spatula. fold the excess baking paper over flat leaving the ends as they are to allow steam to escape. Folding this over will keep your meatloaf tender and moist. Bake in the oven on 170'C/335'F until firm to the touch (approx. 35 – 40 minutes). Open baking paper and bake for a further 5 minutes. Remove from oven and let sit for 5 minutes.

Turn our on a serving platter and slice. Serve with Butter Sautéed broccoli and green beans.

References

References

AACC. (2016). Albumin. Retrieved August 10, 2017, from https://labtestsonline.org/understanding/analytes/albumin/tab/test/

Adam, B., & Rieger, E. (2012). How self-perception , emotion and beliefs influence eating and weight-related behaviour. In R. S. Magnusson, S. M. Twigg, & L. A. Baur (Eds.), *A Modern Epidemic: Expert Perspective on Obesity and Diabetes* (pp. 263–274). Sydney, New South Wales: Sydney University Press.

Allen, F. M., Stillman, E., & Fitz, R. (1919). No Title. New York: The Rockefeller Institute for Medical Research.

Antinori, S., Milazzo, L., Sollima, S., Galli, M., & Corellin, M. (2016). Candidemia and invasive candidiasis in adults: A narrative review. *European Journal of Internal Medicine*, *October*(34), 21–28. Retrieved from https://www.ncbi.nlm.nih.gov/pubmed/27394927

Aranow. MD, C. (2011). Vitamin D and the Immune System. *Journal of Investigative Medicine*, *59*(6), 881–886. https://doi.org/10.231/JIM.0b013e31821b8755.Vitamin

Armour, C., Chaar, B., Murray, M., Ambler, G., & Krass, I. (2012). Current therapies and pharmacy programs for obesity and diabetes. In R. S. Magnusson, L. A. Baur, & S. M. Twigg (Eds.), *A modern epidemic: expert perspectives on obesity and diabetes* (pp. 315–338). Sydney, New South Wales: Sydney University Press.

Arora, S. K., & McFarlane, S. I. (2005). The case for low carbohydrate diets in diabetes management. *Nutr Metab (Lond)*, *2*. https://doi.org/10.1186/1743-7075-2-16

ARUP Consult©. (2017). Inflammatory Bowel Disease - IBD. Retrieved August 16, 2017, from https://arupconsult.com/content/inflammatory-bowel-disease

Ascherio, A., Stampfer, M. J., & Willett, W. C. (1999). Trans Fatty Acids and Coronary Heart Disease. Retrieved May 25, 2013, from http://www.drtimdelivers.com/EEasy122605/Harvardtransfats/transfats.html

Australia, H. (2017). Iron deficiency symptoms. Retrieved July 30, 2017, from https://www.healthdirect.gov.au/iron-deficiency-symptoms

Basu, A., Rhone, M., & Lyons, T. J. (2010). Berries: emerging impact on cardiovascular health. *Nutrition Reviews*, *68*(3), 168–77. https://doi.org/10.1111/j.1753-4887.2010.00273.x

Beattie, J., Crozier, A., & Duthie, G. (2005). Potential Health Benefits of Berries. *Current Nutrition & Food Science*, *1*(1), 71–86. https://doi.org/10.2174/1573401052953294

Bergamo, P. (2003). Fat-soluble vitamin contents and fatty acid composition in organic and conventional Italian dairy products. *Food Chemistry*, *82*(4), 625–631. https://doi.org/10.1016/S0308-8146(03)00036-0

Black Dog Institute. (2013). Mindfulness in everyday life. Randwick NSW. Retrieved from http://www.blackdoginstitute.org.au/docs/10.MindfulnessinEverydayLife.pdf

Boden, G., Sargrad, K., Homko, C., Mozzoli, M., & Stein, T. P. (2005). Effect of a low-carbohydrate diet on appetite, blood glucose levels, and insulin resistance in obese patients with type 2 diabetes. *Ann Intern Med*, *142*. https://doi.org/10.7326/0003-4819-142-6-200503150-00006

Boyer, J., & Liu, R. H. (2004). Apple phytochemicals and their health benefits. *Nutrition Journal*, *3*, 5. https://doi.org/10.1186/1475-2891-3-5

Bragg, C. P., & Bragg, P. (1999). The Miracle of Fasting. Santa Barbara, CA: Health Science.doi.org/10.7326/0003-4819-140-10-200405180-00006

Brand-Miller, J., Hayne, S., Petocz, P., & Colagiuri, S. (2003). Low–Glycemic Index Diets in the Management of Diabetes: A meta-analysis of randomized controlled trials . *Diabetes Care* , *26*(8), 2261–2267. https://doi.org/10.2337/diacare.26.8.2261

Brand-Miller, Jennie, Ambler, & Geoffrey. (2012). Nutrition therapy in the treatment of diabetes. In R. S. Magnusson, S. M. Twigg, & L. A. Baur (Eds.), *A modern epidemic: expert perspectives on obesity and diabetes* (pp. 300–314). Sydney, New South Wales: Sydney University Press. Retrieved from http://apps.isiknowledge.com/full_record.do?prod-uct=UA&search_mode=CombineSearches&qid=6&SID=R2onXPd3iL9fD8YHhQv&page=9&doc=419

Braun, L., & Cohen, M. (2011). *Herbs & Natural Supplements - An Evidence Based Guide* (3rd ed.). Churchill Livingstone Elsevier.

Brenner, D. M., Moeller, M. J., Chey, W. D., & Schoenfeld, P. S. (2009). The Utility of Probiotics in the Treatment of Irritable Bowel Syndrome: A Systematic Review. *The American Journal of Gastroenterology*, *104*(4), 1033–1049. https://doi.org/10.1038/ajg.2009.25

Brown, J. E. (2011). *Nutrition through the Life Cycle* (Fourth). Belmont, California: Cengage Learning. https://doi.org/10.1039/9781847559463

Brugnara, C. (2003). Iron deficiency and erythropoiesis: New diagnostic approaches. *Clinical Chemistry*, *49*(10), 1573–1578. https://doi.org/10.1373/49.10.1573

Bures, J., Cyrany, J., Kohoutova, D., Förstl, M., Rejchrt, S., Kvetina, J., … Kopacova, M. (2010). Small intestinal bacterial overgrowth syndrome. *World Journal of Gastroenterology*, *16*(24), 2978–90. https://doi.org/10.3748/wjg.v16.i24.2978

Cagnacci, A. (2003). Relation of homocysteine, folate, and vitamin B12 to bone mineral density of postmenopausal women. *Bone*, *33*(6), 956–959. https://doi.org/10.1016/j.bone.2003.07.001

Carter, S. M., Kerridge, I., Rychetnik, L., & King, L. (2012). The ethical implications of intervening in bodyweight. In R. S. Magnusson, S. M. Twigg, & L. A. Baur (Eds.), *A Modern Epidemic: Expert Perspective on Obesity and Diabetes* (pp. 191–206). Sydney, New South Wales: Sydney University Press.

Centers for Disease Control and Prevention. (2015). Invasive Candidiasis. Retrieved August 7, 2017, from https://www.cdc.gov/fungal/diseases/candidiasis/invasive/

Chaput, J.-P., Després, J.-P., Bouchard, C., & Tremblay, A. (2012). Longer sleep duration associates with lower adiposity gain in adult short sleepers. *International Journal of Obesity*, *36*(5), 752–756. https://doi.org/10.1038/ijo.2011.110

Christos S. Mantzoros, MD, Ds. (Ed.). (2009). *Nutrition and Metabolism: Underlying Mechanisms and Clinical Consequences*. Humana Press, c/o Springer Science + Business Media, LLC, 233 Spring Street, New York, NY 10013, USA.

College, N. R., Walker, B. R., & Ralston, S. H. (2010). *Davidson's Principles and Practice of Medicine*. (N. R. College, B. R. Walker, & S. H. Ralston, Eds.) (21st ed.). Edinburgh London New York Oxford Philadelphia St Louis Sydney Toronto 2010: Elsevier. Retrieved from www.elsevierhealth.com

Cooper, R., Cutler, J., Desvigne-Nickens, P., Fortmann, S. P., Friedman, L., Havlik, R., ... Thom, T. (2000). Trends and Disparities in Coronary Heart Disease, Stroke, and Other Cardiovascular Diseases in the United States : Findings of the National Conference on Cardiovascular Disease Prevention. *Circulation*, *102*(25), 3137–3147. https://doi.org/10.1161/01.CIR.102.25.3137

Croxford, S., Itsiopoulos, C., Forsyth, A., Belski, R., Thodis, A., Shepherd, S., & Tierney, A. (2015). *Food & Nutrition Throughout Life*. (S. Croxford, C. Itsiopoulos, A. Forsyth, R. Belski, A. Thodis, S. Shepherd, & A. Tierney, Eds.). Crows Nest, NSW: Allen & Unwin.

Denke, M. A. (2001). Metabolic effects of high-protein, low-carbohydrate diets. *Am J Cardiol*, *88*. https://doi.org/10.1016/S0002-9149(01)01586-7

Diet & Nutrition for Menopause. (n.d.). Retrieved May 1, 2013, from http://www.redhotmamas.org/nutrition-menopause

Durnin, J. V. G. A., & Womersley, J. (1974). Body fat assessed from total body density and its estimation from skinfold thickness: measurements on 481 men and women aged from 16 to 72 years. *Br J Nutr*, *32*. https://doi.org/10.1079/BJN19740060

Encyclopedia Brittanica. (2012). immune system (physiology) : Antibody-mediated immune mechanisms. Retrieved August 23, 2012, from http://www.britannica.com/EBchecked/topic/283636/immune-system/215582/Antibody-mediated-immune-mechanisms

Foodzone. (2013). Sydney, NSW: Digital App Solutions Pty Ltd. Retrieved from https://foodzone.com.au

Fuller, R. (1992). History and development of probiotics. In *Probiotics: The scientific basis* (pp. 1–8). Dordrecht: Springer Netherlands. https://doi.org/10.1007/978-94-011-2364-8_1

Fung, T. T., Rimm, E. B., Spiegelman, D., Rifai, N., Tofler, G. H., Willett, W. C., & Hu, F. B. (2001). Association between dietary patterns and plasma biomarkers of obesity and cardiovascular disease risk. *The American Journal of Clinical Nutrition*, *73*(1), 61–67. Retrieved from http://ajcn.nutrition.org/content/73/1/61.abstract

Gallagher, D., Heymsfield, S. B., Heo, M., Jebb, S. A., Murgatroyd, P. R., & Sakamoto, Y. (2000). Healthy percentage body fat ranges : an approach for developing guidelines based on body mass index 1 – 3. *American Journal of Clinical Nutrition*, (72), 694–701.

Gannon, M. C., & Nuttall, F. Q. (2004). Effect of a high-protein, low-carbohydrate diet on blood glucose control in people with type 2 diabetes. *Diabetes*, *53*. https://doi.org/10.2337/diabetes.53.9.2375

Gasbarrini, A., Lauritano, E. C., Gabrielli, M., Scarpellini, F. Lupascu, À., Ojetti, V., & Gasbarrini, G. (2007). Small Intestinal Bacterial Overgrowth: Diagnosis and Treatment. *Digestive Diseases*, *25*(3), 237–240. https://doi.org/10.1159/000103892

Gasche, C., Berstad, A., Befrits, R., Beglinger, C., Dignass, A., Erichsen, K., ... Van Assche, G. (2007). Guidelines on the diagnosis and management of iron deficiency and anemia in inflammatory bowel diseases. *Inflammatory Bowel Diseases*, *13*(12), 1545–1553. https://doi.org/10.1002/ibd.20285

German, J. B., & Dillard, C. J. (2006). Composition, structure and absorption of milk lipids: a source of energy, fat-soluble nutrients and bioactive molecules. *Critical Reviews in Food Science and Nutrition*, *46*(1), 57–92. https://doi.org/10.1080/10408690590957098

Gottschall, E. (2004). *Breaking the Vicious Cycle - Intestinal Health Through Diet* (Rev. ed. o). Ontario, Canada: Kirkton Press Ltd.

Gropper, S. S., & Smith, J. L. (2013). *Advanced Nutrition and Human Metabolism* (6th ed.). Wadsworth: Cengage Learning.

Gutierrez-Repiso, C., Soriguer, F., Rubio-Martn, E., Esteva de Antonio, I., Ruiz de Adana, M. S., Almaraz, M. C., ... Rojo-Martinez, G. (2014). Night-time sleep duration and the incidence of obesity and type 2 diabetes. Findings from the prospective Pizarra study. *Sleep Medicine*, *15*(11), 1398–1404. https://doi.org/10.1016/j.sleep.2014.06.014

Halton, T. L., Willett, W. C., Liu, S., Manson, J. E., Stampfer, M. J., & Hu, F. B. (2006). Potato and french fry consumption and risk of type 2 diabetes in women. *The American Journal of Clinical Nutrition*, *83*(2), 284–290. Retrieved from http://ajcn.nutrition.org/content/83/2/284.abstract

Hasler, C. M. (1998). Functional Foods: Their Role in Disease Prevention and Health Promotion. Retrieved May 25, 2013, from http://www.nutriwatch.org/04Foods/ff.html

Hayes, S. C., Hayes, S. C., Jacobson, N. S., Follette, V. M., & Dougher, M. J. (1994). *Acceptance and change: content and context in psychotherapy*. (null, Ed.) (Vol. null).

Hayes, S. C., Strosahl, K. D., & Wilson, K. G. (1999). *Acceptance and commitment therapy: an experiential approach to behavior change*. (null, Ed.) (Vol. null).

Health Direct Australia. (2017). Iron deficiency symptoms. Retrieved July 30, 2017, from https://www.healthdirect.gov.au/iron-deficiency-symptoms

Horne, B. D., Muhlestein, J. B., & Anderson, J. L. (2015). Health effects of intermittent fasting: hormesis or harm? A systematic review. *The American Journal of Clinical Nutrition*, *102*(2), 464–70. https://doi.org/10.3945/ajcn.115.109553

Hu, F. B. (2003). Plant-based foods and prevention of cardiovascular disease: an overview. *The American Journal of Clinical Nutrition* , *78*(3), 544S–551S. Retrieved from http://ajcn.nutrition.org/content/78/3/544S.abstract

Intensive blood-glucose control with sulphonylureas or insulin compared with conventional treatment and risk of complications in patients with type 2 diabetes (UKPDS 33). UK Prospective Diabetes Study (UKPDS) Group. (1998). *Lancet*, *352*. https://doi.org/10.1016/S0140-6736(98)07019-6

Iveson, C. (2002). Solution-focused brief therapy. *Advances in Psychiatric Treatment*, *8*(2). Retrieved from http://apt.rcpsych.org/content/8/2/149

Jenkins, D. J. A., Kendall, C. W. C., Marchie, A., Parker, T. L., Connelly, P. W., Qian, W., … Spiller, G. A. (2002). Dose Response of Almonds on Coronary Heart Disease Risk Factors: Blood Lipids, Oxidized Low-Density Lipoproteins, Lipoprotein(a), Homocysteine, and Pulmonary Nitric Oxide: A Randomized, Controlled, Crossover Trial . *Circulation* , *106*(11), 1327–1332. https://doi.org/10.1161/01.CIR.0000028421.91733.20

Jeukendrup, A., & Gleeson, M. (2010). *Sports Nutrition: An Introduction to Energy Production and Performance* (Second). Champaign, IL: Human Kinetics.

Juranić, Z., & Žižak, Ž. (2005). Biological activities of berries: From antioxidant capacity to anti-cancer effects. *BioFactors*, *23*(4), 207–211. Retrieved from http://iospress.metapress.com/content/528QHLJ6T7X052M5

Kabat-Zinn, J., Goleman, D., & Gurin, J. (1993). *Mind/body medicine*. (null, Ed.) (Vol. null).

Katan, M. B. (2006). Regulation of trans fats: the gap, the Polder, and McDonald's French fries. *Atherosclerosis. Supplements*, *7*(2), 63–6. https://doi.org/10.1016/j.atherosclerosissup.2006.04.013

http://www.kefir.net/sources/ Benefits of Kefir

Kerr, M., & Cafasso, J. (2017). Malabsorption Syndrome. Retrieved August 10, 2017, from http://www.healthline.com/health/malabsorption#complications7

Klein, S., Sheard, N. F., Pi-Sunyer, S., Daly, A., Wylie-Rosett, J., Kulkarni, K., & Clark, N. G. (2004). Weight management through lifestyle modification for the prevention and management of type 2 diabetes: rationale and strategies. A statement of the American Diabetes Association, the North American Association for the Study of Obesity, and the American So. *Am J Clin Nutr*, *80*.

Kossoff, E. H., & Hartman, A. L. (2012). Ketogenic diets: new advances for metabolism-based therapies. *Current Opinion In Neurology*, *25*(2), 173–178. https://doi.org/10.1097/WCO.0b013e3283515e4a

Lethem, J. (2002). Brief Solution Focused Therapy. *Child and Adolescent Mental Health*, *7*(4), 189–192. https://doi.org/10.1111/1475-3588.00033

Liu, S. (2002). Intake of Refined Carbohydrates and Whole Grain Foods in Relation to Risk of Type 2 Diabetes Mellitus and Coronary Heart Disease. *Journal of the American College of Nutrition* , *21*(4), 298–306. Retrieved from http://www.jacn.org/content/21/4/298.abstract

Magee, L., & Hale, L. (2012). Longitudinal associations between sleep duration and subsequent weight gain: A systematic review. *Sleep Medicine Reviews*, *16*(3), 231–241. https://doi.org/10.1016/j.smrv.2011.05.005

Magnusson, R. S. (2012). Expert perspectives on obesity and diabetes. In *A modern epidemic: expert perspectives on obesity and diabetes*.

Magnusson, R. S. (2012). How law and regulation can add value to prevention strategies for obesity and diabetes. In R. S. Magnusson, S. M. Twigg, & L. A. Baur (Eds.), *A modern epidemic: Expert perspectives on obesity and diabetes* (pp. 207–244). Sydney, New South Wales: Sydney University Press.

Maguire, L. S., O'Sullivan, S. M., Galvin, K., O'Connor, T. P., & O'Brien, N. M. (2004). Fatty acid profile, tocopherol, squalene and phytosterol content of walnuts, almonds, peanuts, hazelnuts and the macadamia nut. *International Journal of Food Sciences and Nutrition*, *55*(3), 171–8. https://doi.org/10.1080/09637480410001725175

Mahan, L. K., Escott-Stump, S., & Raymond, J. L. (2012). *Krause's Food and the Nutrition Care Process* (13th ed.). Elsevier.

McGill, M., & Overland, J. (2012). Diabetes healthcare strategies to cope with the growing epidemic. In R. S. Magnusson, S. M. Twigg, & L. A. Baur (Eds.), *Modern Epidemic: Expert Perspectives on Obesity and Diabetes* (pp. 339–352). Sydney, New South Wales: Sydney University Press.

Meckling, K. A., O'Sullivan, C., & Saari, D. (2004). Comparison of a low-fat diet to a low-carbohydrate diet on weight loss, body composition, and risk factors for diabetes and cardiovascular disease in free-living, overweight men and women. *J Clin Endocrinol Metab*, *89*. https://doi.org/10.1210/jc.2003-031606

Melbourne Academic Mindfulness Interest Group. (2006). Mindfulness-based psychotherapies: a review of conceptual foundations, empirical evidence and practical considerations. *Australian and New Zealand Journal of Psychiatry*, *40*(4), 285–294. https://doi.org/10.1080/j.1440-1614.2006.01794.x

Melnik, B. C. (2009). Milk--the promoter of chronic Western diseases. *Medical Hypotheses*, *72*(6), 631–9. https://doi.org/10.1016/j.mehy.2009.01.008

Miller, W. R., & Rollnick, S. (2002). *Motivational Interviewing:*

Mitchell, A., & Cormack, M. (1998). *The Therapeutic Relationship in Complementary Health Care*. London: Elselvier Limited.

Mudd, J. E., Mccollum, E. E., Rosen, K. H., & Stith, S. M. (2000). *Solution-Focused Therapy and Communication Skills Training : An integrated approach to couples therapy*. Virginia Polytechnic Institute and State University in, Blacksburg, Virginia.

National Institutes of Health. (2012). Calculate Your BMI - Metric BMI Calculator. Retrieved September 17, 2012, from http://www.nhlbisupport.com/bmi/bmi-m.htm

Natural Standard - Nutritional deficiencies. (n.d.). Retrieved March 27, 2012, from http://www.naturalstandard.com.ezproxy.endeavour.edu.au:2048/databases/environment/condition nutritionaldeficiencies.asp

Nielsen, J. V, Jonsson, E., & Nilsson, A. K. (2005). Lasting improvement of hyperglycaemia and bodyweight: low-carbohydrate diet in type 2 diabetes. A brief report. *Ups J Med Sci, 110*.

Organic Facts. (2017). 9 Wonderful Benefits of Pistachios. Retrieved from https://www.organicfacts.net/health-benefits/seed-and-nut/health-benefits-of-pistachio.html

Orsillo, S. M., Roemer, L., Lerner, J. B., Tull, M. T., Hayes, S. C., Follette, V. M., & Linehan, M. M. (2004). *Mindfulness and acceptance: expanding the cognitive-behavioral tradition*. (null, Ed.) (Vol. null).

Osler, W., & McCrae, T. (1923). No Title. New York: Appleton and Co.

Pagana, K. D., & Pagana, T. J. (2013). *Mosby's Manual of Diagnostic and Laboratory Tests* (Fifth). St Louis, Missouri: Elsevier - Health Sciences Division.

Patel, S. R., Hayes, A. L., Blackwell, T., Evans, D. S., Ancoli-Israel, S., Wing, Y. K., & Stone, K. L. (2014). The association between sleep patterns and obesity in older adults. *International Journal of Obesity, 38*(9), 1159–1164. https://doi.org/10.1038/ijo.2014.13

Phongsavan, P., Rissel, C., King, L., & Bauman, A. (2012). Whole of society approaches to preventing obesity and diabetes. In R. S. Magnusson, S. M. Twigg, & L. A. Baur (Eds.), *A Modern Epidemic: Expert Perspective on Obesity and Diabetes* (pp. 245–259). Sydney, New South Wales: Sydney University Press.

Pitchford, P. (2002). *Healing With Whole Foods: Asian Traditions and Modern Nutrition* (Third). Berkeley, Caifornia: North Atlantic Books.

Prietl, B., Treiber, G., Pieber, T. R., & Amrein, K. (2013). Vitamin D and Immune Function. *Practical Diabetes, 5*(7), 2502–2521. https://doi.org/10.3390/nu5072502

Prospective Studies Collaboration. (2009). Body-mass index and cause-specifi c mortality in 900 000 adults : collaborative analyses of 57 prospective. *The Lancet, 373*(9669), 1083–1096. https://doi.org/10.1016/S0140-6736(09)60318-4

Purnell, J. Q., Hokanson, J. E., Marcovina, S. M., Steffes, M. W., Cleary, P. A., & Brunzell, J. D. (1998). Effect of excessive weight gain with intensive therapy of type 1 diabetes on lipid levels and blood pressure: results from the DCCT. Diabetes Control and Complications Trial. *JAMA, 280*. https://doi.org/10.1001/jama.280.2.140

Raik, E. (2004). Coeliac disease. *Common Sense Pathology*, (June), 1–7.

Reeves, G. (2007). Abnormal laboratory results: C-reactive protein. *Australian Prescriber, 30*(3), 74–76. https://doi.org/10.18773/austprescr.2007.043

Rolfes, S. R., Pinna, K., & Whitney, E. (2009a). Anthopometric Data. In A. Lustig & E. Feldman (Eds.), *Understanding Normal and Clinical Nutrition* (eighth, p. 599). Belmont California: Yolanda Cossio.

Rolfes, S. R., Pinna, K., & Whitney, E. (2009b). Energy Balance and Body Composition. In A. Lustig & E. Feldman (Eds.), *Understanding Normal and Clinical Nutrition* (Eighth, p. 259). Belmont, California: Yolanda Cossio.

Samaha, F. F., Iqbal, N., Seshadri, P., Chicano, K., Daily, D., McGrory, J., … Stern, L. (2003). A low-carbohydrate as compared with a low-fat diet in severe obesity. *N Engl J Med, 348*. https://doi.org/10.1056/NEJMoa022637

Sanders, T., & Emery, P. (2003). *Molecular Basis of Human Nutrition*. Nutrition. London: Taylor and Francis.

Sapse, A. T. (1997). Cortisol, high cortisol diseases and anti-cortisol therapy. *Psychoneuroendocrinology*. https://doi.org/10.1016/S0306-4530(97)00024-3

Sarris, J., & Wardle, J. (2010). *Clinical Naturopathy - An Evidence Based Guide to Practice*. Churchill Livingstone Elsevier.

Sharman, M. J., Gomez, A. L., Kraemer, W. J., & Volek, J. S. (2004). Very low-carbohydrate and low-fat diets affect fasting lipids and postprandial lipemia differently in overweight men. *J Nutr, 134*.

Sheard, N. F., Clark, N. G., Brand-Miller, J. C., Franz, M. J., Pi-Sunyer, F. X., Mayer-Davis, E., … Geil, P. (2004). Dietary Carbohydrate (Amount and Type) in the Prevention and Management of Diabetes: A statement by the American Diabetes Association . *Diabetes Care , 27*(9), 2266–2271. https://doi.org/10.2337/diacare.27.9.2266

Smout, M. (2012). Acceptance and commitment therapy. *Australian Family Physician, 41Asia Pacific Journal of Clinical Nutrition, 14*(2), 120–130.

Vernon, M. C., Mavropoulos, J., Yancy, W. S., & Westman, E. C. (2003). Brief report: clinical experience of a carbohydrate-restricted diet: effect on diabetes mellitus. *Metabolic Syndrome and Related Disorders, 1*. https://doi.org/10.1089/154041903322716714

Volek, J. S., Sharman, M. J., Gomez, A. L., DiPasquale, C., Roti, M., Pumerantz, A., & Kraemer, W. J. (2004). Comparison of a very low-carbohydrate and low-fat diet on fasting lipids, LDL subclasses, insulin resistance, and postprandial lipemic responses in overweight women. *J Am Coll Nutr, 23*. https://

Størsrud, S., Hulthén, L. R., & Lenner, R. A. (2007). Beneficial effects of oats in the gluten-free diet of adults with special reference to nutrient status, symptoms and subjective experiences. *British Journal of Nutrition*, 90(1), 101. https://doi.org/10.1079/BJN2003872

Sweeney, T. E., & Morton, J. M. (2013). The Human Gut Microbiome. *JAMA Surgery*, 148(6), 563. https://doi.org/10.1001/jamasurg.2013.5

Tamparo, C. D., & Lindh, W. Q. (2012). *Therapeutic Communications for Health Care* (Fourth). Boston: Cengage Learning. Retrieved from https://books.google.com.au/books?id=AeMIAAAAQBAJ

The Atkins Trial Kit Handbook: A Simple Guide to Doing Atkins. (2001). Ronkonkoma, NY: Atkins Nutritionals, Inc.

The World Health Organization (WHO). (2008). *Waist Circumference and Waist-Hip Ratio Report of a WHO Expert Consultation*. Geneva, Switzerland.

Toledo, P., Andrén, A., & Björck, L. (2002). Composition of raw milk from sustainable production systems. *International Dairy Journal*, 12(1), 75–80. https://doi.org/10.1016/S0958-6946(01)00148-0

Twigg, S. M., & Mclennan, S. V. (2012). 20 Managing diabetes complications in the clinical arena. In R. S. Magnusson, S. M. Twigg, & L. A. Baur (Eds.), *A modern epidemic: expert perspectives on obesity and diabetes* (pp. 353–371). Sydney, New South Wales: Sydney University Press.

Vattem, D. A., Ghaedian, R., & Shetty, K. (2005). Enhancing health benefits of berries through phenolic antioxidant enrichment: focus on cranberry. *Asia Pacific Journal of Clinical Nutrition*, 14(2), 120–130.

Vernon, M. C., Mavropoulos, J., Yancy, W. S., & Westman, E. C. (2003). Brief report: clinical experience of a carbohydrate-restricted diet: effect on diabetes mellitus. *Metabolic Syndrome and Related Disorders*, 1. https://doi.org/10.1089/154041903322716714

Volek, J. S., Sharman, M. J., Gomez, A. L., DiPasquale, C., Roti, M., Pumerantz, A., & Kraemer, W. J. (2004). Comparison of a very low-carbohydrate and low-fat diet on fasting lipids, LDL subclasses, insulin resistance, and postprandial lipemic responses in overweight women. *J Am Coll Nutr*, 23. https://doi.org/10.1080/07315724.2004.10719359

Volek, J. S., Sharman, M. J., Love, D. M., Avery, N. G., Gomez, A. L., Scheett, T. P., & Kraemer, W. J. (2002). Body composition and hormonal responses to a carbohydrate-restricted diet. *Metabolism*, 51. https://doi.org/10.1053/meta.2002.32037

Wachtel, P. L. (2011). *Therapeutic Communication: Knowing what to Say When* (Second). Guilford Publications. Retrieved from https://books.google.com.au/books?id=kW6NRZkfjZIC

Wahlqvist, M. (2011). Functional Foods. In *Food & Nutrition: Food and Health Systems in Australia And New Zealand* (3rd Editio, pp. 184–186). Crows Nest, NSW.

Walsh, R., Scotton, B. W., Chinen, A. B., & Battista, J. R. (1996). *Textbook of transpersonal psychiatry and psychology*. (null, Ed.) (Vol. null).

Webster-Gandy, J., Madden, A., & Holdsworth, M. (2006). *Oxford Handbook of Nutrition and Dietetics*. Oxford, New York: Oxford University Press, Inc. https://doi.org/10.1017/CBO9781107415324.004

Weight-loss Plan For Pre-diabetes | LIVESTRONG.COM. (n.d.). Retrieved October 21, 2012, from http://www.livestrong.com/article/427586-weight-loss-plan-for-pre-diabetes/

Westcoast Integrative Health. (2015). What Causes SIBO? – Psychiatry. Retrieved August 13, 2017, from http://sibotesting.com/what-causes-sibo-psychiatry/

Westman, E. C., Yancy, W. S., Edman, J. S., Tomlin, K. F., & Perkins, C. E. (2002). Effect of six-month adherence to a very-low-carbohydrate diet program. *Am J Med*, 113. https://doi.org/10.1016/S0002-9343(02)01129-4

Whitney, E. N., Cataldo, C. B., & Rolfes, S. R. (1983). *Understanding Normal & Clinical Nutrition*. (P. A. Lewis, Ed.) (Fouth Edit). St. Paul: West Publishing Company.

Wilson, K. G., Murrell, A. R., Hayes, S. C., Follette, V. M., & Linehan, M. M. (2004). *Mindfulness and acceptance: expanding the cognitive-behavioral tradition*. (null, Ed.) (Vol. null).

Xiao, Q., Arem, H., Moore, S. C., Hollenbeck, A. R., & Matthews, C. E. (2013). A large prospective investigation of sleep duration,weight change, and obesity in the NIH-AARP diet and health study cohort. *American Journal of Epidemiology*, 178(11), 1600–1610. https://doi.org/10.1093/aje/kwt180

Yancy, W. S., & Boan, J. (2005). Adherence to Diet Recommendations. Mahwah, NJ: Lawrence Erlbaum Associates, Inc.

Yancy, W. S., Foy, M., Chalecki, A. M., Vernon, M. C., & Westman, E. C. (2005). A low-carbohydrate, ketogenic diet to treat type 2 diabetes. *Nutrition & Metabolism*, 2(1), 34. https://doi.org/10.1186/1743-7075-2-34

Yancy, W. S., Olsen, M. K., Guyton, J. R., Bakst, R. P., & Westman, E. C. (2004). A low-carbohydrate, ketogenic diet versus a low-fat diet to treat obesity and hyperlipidemia: a randomized, controlled trial. *Ann Intern Med*, 140. https://doi.org/10.7326/0003-4819-140-10-200405180-00006

Yancy, W. S., Vernon, M. C., & Westman, E. C. (2003). Brief report: a pilot trial of a low-carbohydrate, ketogenic diet in patients with type II diabetes. *Metabolic Syndrome and Related Disorders*, 1. https://doi.org/10.1089/154041903322716723

What is Kefir http://www.bodyandsoul.com.au/nutrition/nutrition-tips/what-is-kefir-the-benefits-of-this-wonder-drink/news-story/ef481ed0a18400d59d3e2aa8dcf0058a

Notes

Notes

- THIS PAGE HAS BEEN INTENTIONALLY LEFT BLANK -

Transition into Balance after Reset

Do you want to adopt a way of eating that is **low-carb, ketosis inducing, but non restrictive and full of variety?**

Establish healthy balanced intake targets to promote ongoing weight loss and well being - advocating variety, wholefoods and being human!

ALL IN ONE COMPLETE PROGRAM PACKAGE
"Balanced Macros - The Complete Solution to Bariatric Keto"

Designed by Holistic Nutritionist Carrie Ross, to help post-op bariatric clients establish appropriate food portioning, scheduling and adequate nutritional intakes.

What must be understood about the post-bariatric digestive system is that

IT IS ABOUT QUALITY AS IT CAN NO-LONGER BE ABOUT QUANTITY!

HOW DO YOU DO IT?

1. Get Your Balanced Macros Official program eBook which contains:
* Program Outlines and Healthy Habit Guidelines * Positive Affirmation/ Self Assessment thought pages * 8-Different Example Menus * Balanced Macros Snack and Meal Cheat Sheets * Low-Carb/ Balanced Macro Food lists * Tips and Tricks for Surviving Social events and Holiday * Gut health and Bariatric Vitamin suggestion * Printable Food-Diary Journal Pages * Recipes and More...*

2. Get Your Personalised Macronutrient Profile Report
Formulated macros to work with, designed specifically for you.

3. The Deliciously Low-Carb Cook eBook
*Yours to download and keep and put to good use with your new Macros *

4. Additional Health and Lifestyle Coaching Sheets
Dependant on needs.

5. Ongoing Access to a Live Vibrant Community of Bariatric Peers..
That doesn't just claim to hold your hand and be supportive,
it actually does !!

The unique Balanced Macros protocol is unlike any other program and your ongoing success is OUR GOAL, with full support and guidance.

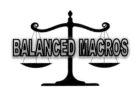

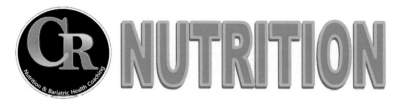

Balanced Macros Program©

The Complete Solution to Bariatric Keto

Non Restrictive Dietary Design
For any stage of your weight loss journey

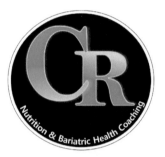

Find Us on Facebook

CR NUTRITION & BARIATRIC HEALTH COACHING

www.crnutrition.net

Manufactured by Amazon.ca
Bolton, ON

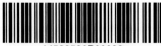